Managed Care
practice and progress

Robert Royce

Head of Policy/Secretary
Dyfed Powys Health Authority

Radcliffe Medical Press

© 1997 Robert Royce

Radcliffe Medical Press Ltd
18 Marcham Road, Abingdon, Oxon OX14 1AA, UK

Radcliffe Medical Press, Inc.
141 Fifth Avenue, New York, NY 10010, USA

British Library Cataloguing in Publication Data

A catalogue record for this book is available from the British Library.

ISBN 1 85775 280 5

Library of Congress Cataloging-in-Publication Data is available.

Typeset by Advance Typesetting Ltd, Oxon
Printed and bound in Great Britain by Redwood Books, Trowbridge, Wiltshire

Contents

Preface

I wrote this book initially with the sole intention of giving readers an in-depth appreciation of managed care in the USA and a balanced assessment of its applicability to the UK. As time passed it became obvious that, in addition to the above, I was being drawn to comment about the current state of the NHS reforms, and that this would give greater focus to observations about US health care, management and techniques. My consistent aim has been to produce a work that would add to most readers' knowledge and will contribute to the development of health care management regardless of which party occupies government, and which path reform takes.

I was able to write this book from first-hand experience of the managed care industry, via a six-month secondment to Sentara Health System in Virginia, USA – one of the leading health care companies on the East Coast. I am extremely grateful to Sentara for the unparalleled access to meetings, documents and personnel afforded to me during my time there. The secondment was made possible by the support of the then chief executive of Dyfed Health Authority – Mike Ponton – and formed part of the leadership development programme for NHS Wales. I strongly believe that it is extremely important that the NHS encourages external placements as a way of developing its staff, and encouraging access to new ideas. Insularity is one of the public sector's most enduring and least attractive characteristics.

Amongst the many individuals I wish to thank for their assistance in getting this book written and making my time in the USA so productive are Richard Hill, Ted Willie, Tommy Lee, Bert Reese, Bob Rash, and Anne Marie and John Cochrane (in the USA), and Mike Ponton, Sue Brown and David Evans (in the UK). Finally, I wish to thank my wife – Jill – for her unrelenting understanding and support. The views in this book are the author's and should not be seen as representing that of his employer – Dyfed Powys Health Authority – or NHS Wales. In the course of this book the terms 'physician' and 'doctor' are used interchangeably as are the terms 'HMO' and 'managed care'. A glossary is provided on pages 210–223.

Robert Royce
December 1996

Abbreviations

ADS	Alternative delivery system
ALOS	Average length of stay
CABG	Coronary artery bypass graft
CMDS	Contracting minimum data set
CPN	Community psychiatric nurse
CT	Computerized tomography
DNR	Do not resuscitate
EC	European Community
ECR	Extra contractual referral
EIS	Executive information system
GPFH	General practitioner fundholder
HEDIS	Health plan employer data and information set
HISS	Hospital information support system
HMO	Health maintenance organization
IPA	Independent practice association
IT	Information technology
ITU	Intensive treatment units
LOS	Length of stay
MIS	Management information system
MPV	Medical practice variation
MRI	Magnetic resonance imaging
MTD	Month to date
NCQA	National Council for Quality Accreditation
PAS	Patient administration system
PCP	Primary care physician
PFI	Private finance initiative
PPO	Preferred provider organization
SHP	Sentara Health Plan
UR	Utilization review
WLI	Waiting list initiative
WTE	Whole time equivalent
YTD	Year to date

Why study managed care?

Most countries are dealing with health care reform as if each was on Mars. Few have tried to learn from others. This indifference to the international face of doctoring is a mistake.

The Economist – July 1991

Any writer on health care in the USA has to overcome the natural inclination to concentrate on the differences with the British National Health Service (NHS), which can quickly lead to the erroneous conclusion that we can learn nothing of value from this complex, fragmented and expensive industry. The use of the term 'industry' is deliberate and is meant to convey both the financial sums involved, and the management techniques and operating philosophies displayed by those working within it. It remains unfashionable to think of the NHS in such terms, but this book sets out to demonstrate that both systems share certain common concerns – and that this is particularly true when looking at the role and methodologies used by managed care companies in general, and health maintenance organizations (HMOs) in particular. It should also be borne in mind that the US health care system has operated in a market environment for many years. As a result it has developed some advanced micro-management techniques and an operating philosophy dominated by the knowledge that patients can – and often will – move company/provider if they are dissatisfied with the service they receive and/or consider it too expensive. Only those married to the most rigid of preconceptions as to what constitutes 'good health care' would consider such experience irrelevant to the UK.

Notwithstanding the above, the US health care system exhibits a curious mixture of sophisticated clinical/management techniques and rudimentary omissions. The production and use of information demonstrates a similar inconsistency – but as one might suspect there is a certain internal logic. Systems, reports, ways of managing – and particularly the manner in which health care is delivered (or not delivered in certain circumstances) – are direct responses to the way the US system is structured (sic) and operates. To the outside observer this represents a potentially rich, but also confusing environment from which to learn: particularly when the objective is to utilize that which is innovative and transferable and reject the less desirable features of what is widely (and rightly) seen as a flawed system.

With this in mind this book examines the principal methods by which managed care in the USA operates and considers its relevance to the embryonic NHS 'internal market'. Strengths and weaknesses are identified in each health care system and areas are highlighted where adoption of new techniques and methods would enhance services in the UK without unduly undermining the basis on which the NHS operates. It is the underlying premise of this book (and indeed of the author's secondment from the NHS which provided much of the reference material and allowed this book to be written) that there are elements of 'foreign' health care systems which can usefully be applied to the UK without the abandonment or undermining of the operating principles of the NHS.

The book also looks at the way one US health care company – Sentara Health System – has developed its managed care business and the direction in which its products are moving, as a means of illustrating models and ideas in circulation. The opportunity is also taken to make some observations about management cultures, and the question is posed as to whether the NHS can hope to obtain the leverage of an effective market (which by no means presupposes an unbridled market system) with its existing management culture, regulations and mindsets.

Managed care: a product of history?

The brief historical overview provided below attempts to show that different systems, with very distinctive features, can end up facing similar issues. Historically, the insurance market in the USA had been relatively indifferent to the manner by which care was provided. Whilst premiums more than covered costs, it kept itself at arm's length from health care delivery – a relationship encouraged by bodies such as the American Medical Association (AMA), which remains fiercely protective of the medical community's professional autonomy.

Although the USA has had the unenviable lead in medical cost inflation for some time, the UK has not escaped from the cost implications of third-party reimbursement for health services (primarily through general taxation) and the enthusiasm with which providers offer, and patients consume, expensive health care. However, payers in both countries are today demanding more control over costs, better quality care, accountability from providers, and fiscally sound and efficient management. In the USA managed care has grown in response to this environment. Part of the UK's response was the creation of the 'internal market'[1,2] in the late 1980s (which is examined later in this chapter).

One subtle difference between the UK and the USA lies in the relative influence of the bodies shaping health care. Unsurprisingly, in both countries government has a significant role to play, but it has been much more central to UK developments than has been the case with its US counterpart. Although the federal government is the largest single purchaser of health services in the USA, many assert that it is the large employers who are the most important influence in shaping health care today (particularly given the failure of the Clinton administration to get its health reforms through Congress). Thus the Health Insurance Association of America[3] can state that:

> Employers as a group constitute an extremely influential element in the evolution of health policy because they are the nation's major purchasers of health benefits. Their preferences will continue to determine developments in managed care.

Although the employer's influence may be in danger of being overstated, it helps to explain the diversity of systems being experimented with in the USA – and their associated strengths and weaknesses.

Notwithstanding the above, there is a continuing debate over the ability of 'market forces' to reform adequately the US health care system (and the UK's for that matter). Reform in this context is usually taken to mean a process which will lead to reduced costs and improved access with no significant reduction in quality of care. Some observers are confident that a dynamic combination of large managed care organizations, employers and politicians harnessing the 'market' will bring about such reform in America. Others – the author included – are more sceptical, believing that the current 'structure' of the US health care system mitigates against fundamental reform and has a natural bias to fragmented and costly service provision. In such an environment a wholesale reliance on the application of market principles to bring about the desired changes is likely to disappoint, not least because markets in health care are so distorted even at the theoretical level – inadequate information, natural monopolies, poor principles of substitution, etc. – as to be inadequate for the desired purpose even before the power of special interest groups, and the particular priorities a society places on the way health care is provided are taken into account.

The author believes that fundamental change of the US health care system – universal coverage, dramatic reductions in administrative and medical costs – will require some form of government (or at the very least state) legislation. The prospects for this are not necessarily encouraging. An oft-heard observation is that there is simply too much money to be made out of the current system, with too many powerful groups benefiting, to allow meaningful reform to take place. Moreover, extending the role of government is always a controversial area for Americans – particularly when the existing regulatory framework and proposed reform packages have a justified reputation both for hypertrophied and impenetrable bureaucracy. This scepticism was expressed in the following passage in the *New York Times*:[4]

> I see people acting like retroviruses. Government regulators, for example, subvert the country's 'immune system' with their excessive diligence. You might think of the regulatory system as being overly protective and becoming the equivalent of an autoimmune disease.

There is another dynamic at work which transcends national borders and is likely to frustrate the cost-containment ambitions of all governments: the current emphasis within western culture on research and development, and improving technology to improve quality of life. A greater reliance on a competitive market may restrict the rate of total spending (although a good case can also be made for such a model accelerating expenditure in this regard) but it will be unable to reverse this trend, whilst there remains a desire and commitment to extend the frontiers of knowledge literally to 'cheat death'. This area is further explored in Chapter 8.

In the meantime the competition currently taking place in the USA is enough to satisfy many employers that they are getting a reasonable deal whilst retaining the choice so many employees see as important. It is in this environment that managed care companies operate, and which is a significant factor towards explaining a structure which to the average UK reader looks bloated, expensive and inherently wasteful in parts. Yet significant inroads could be made to reduce transaction costs and profit margins if some of the major employer groups and health care companies formed strong strategic alliances. One initiative would be to enforce *de facto* industrial standards for uniform billing and use of compatible information systems, and the case for such initiatives should become apparent when these topics are discussed later in the book. The industry needs to make inroads in these areas if it seriously wishes to self-regulate itself and avoid change by government decree.

In the UK, on the other hand, government-initiated concerns have taken centre stage – although from an initial mindset not too dissimilar from that of the insurers. The net result has been the desire to develop systems aimed at controlling costs and assuring quality, enhancing accountability etc., whilst promoting choice – without it seems much awareness that in health care the latter sits in some tension to the cost-control objective.

However, it would seem reasonable to conclude that the NHS has significant in-built advantages and a considerable lead in tackling most of these issues by virtue of its public funding base, history of relative frugality, and unitary structure (compared with the USA). Yet both countries are not short of critics declaring their respective health care systems as being in crisis. If anything, the NHS is the object of the most concern with predictions of financial meltdown,[5] and professional despair being commonplace. Meanwhile, the average American, whilst perhaps prepared to concede the intellectual case for a national health service, would consider its restraints on freedom of choice to be unacceptable – and at odds with both economic and social conventional wisdom in the USA.

From what has been written above, it is clear that the UK cannot afford to be complacent about its system of health care. History shows that organizations need to retain flexibility so as to be able to respond to a changing society's demands, enhance their value and progress – or risk eventual extinction. The NHS and its political masters are currently struggling to reconcile its philosophical roots with the challenges and advantages derived from the introduction of a market forces dynamic. Moreover, in a number of critical areas there remains an ever-widening gap between the objectives management are set and the methods they are allowed to employ to reach them. The techniques and ideas described in this book will not of themselves ease that contradiction but it may help to break down the cultural isolationism which helps limit our possible responses to the challenges we set ourselves.

What then is of value in the managed care experience to the UK? When authors describe developments in managed care, phrases such as 'varied', 'innovative' and 'encouraging' are used, as are terms like 'emerging', 'incomplete' and 'fragmented'. It is in the inherently dynamic and innovative nature of HMO operations (set within a tradition of operating in a market environment) that we may be able to find ideas and techniques to build on to the NHS's inherent strengths and fragile purchaser–provider relationship. The history behind the NHS's current organizational structures is outlined below, so that the likely value and impact of the managed care movement will become apparent.

In 1991 the Conservative government, headed by Margaret Thatcher, launched the NHS into an era of upheaval paralleled only at the time of its creation in 1946. There is precious little sense that this era of sustained turbulence is drawing to a close. Outlined initially in the White Paper *Working for Patients*[1] and subsequently passed into legislation[2] was a series of ideas and reforms which set out to establish an 'internal market' – a formal separation between purchasers and providers.

The contrast with the abortive Clinton Health Plan could not be more stark in terms of process, content and outcome. As the satirist PJ O'Rourke[6] noted: 'The plan is 1400 pages long, detailed specifics to come ... and says the President, this might not be the real or final plan because he's an open-minded guy and wants to be bipartisan and hasn't had a chance to get everybody's input'.

In contrast, *Working for Patients* was pithy to the point of raising (justified) concern that what was being set out was less a blueprint than a haphazard collection of sketches. This was partly confirmed in the diaries[7] of Alan Clark, ex-Conservative minister of defence, in a passage about John Moore, who had been dropped from the government in 1989 after three years as social security secretary:

> During the high months of his status as her [Thatcher's] chosen successor, he framed the Health Service reforms exactly on the basis of what he thought she wanted. But she kept changing her mind. One minute she wanted to go further, the next she got an attack of the doubts, wanted to trim a bit. Each time the unfortunate John agreed, made the adjustments, came back for approval. The result was a total hotchpotch and she ended up thinking he was a wanker, and got rid of him.

Thatcher had announced a review of the NHS in the late 1980s in response to a now-familiar set of problems besetting the service – funding difficulties, too few intensive treatment unit (ITU) beds, adverse media reports – and whatever the dynamics of the internal review process, the end result had two characteristics lacking in its American counterpart:

- it was short, punchy and worked on the principle of setting a direction – details to come later

- it was implemented quickly with no consideration given to establishing pilots and little attention or concession made to its many critics.

The more cynical observer would say that what it did have in common with Clinton's plan was a distinct ambivalence on funding issues (which nevertheless could be said to be at the root of both reform programmes), and a predilection to believe in solutions generated by politicians rather than those actually working in health care.

Chris Ham, writing in the *British Medical Journal*, summed up the government's approach as follows:[8]

> Unlike previous reorganisations, the changes introduced by *Working for Patients* were sketched in broad outline only, with many of the most important details missing. This reflected the tight timescale against which the

white paper was prepared and the fact that most of the central ideas in the reforms had been only partially thought through. There has therefore been no overall plan guiding the implementation of the reforms and little sense of where this will ultimately lead. In business school parlance, *Working for Patients* is best described as an emergent strategy. Expressed in more simple language, Ministers have been making it up as they have been going along … Where these changes will take the NHS is unclear, even (or perhaps especially) to those at the heart of government.

It is not the purpose of this book to detail the history of the reforms, but an attempt is made to highlight what its principal characteristics were and where they might be leading. Certainly, it is possible to trace an evolution to 'managed care' similar to the term which Americans understand it to be. Other directions are also possible, and some would argue more likely. At the time of writing (autumn 1996), a general election is due and the question needs to be asked if a Labour victory would spell the end of the reform process in general and the internal market in particular.

We can try and answer this by examining the current state of the Conservative government's reforms. Coincidentally, this should highlight key differences with the USA and what opportunities there might be for managed care techniques to make inroads within the NHS.

The first point to be made is that the 1991 act made no changes to the principles by which UK residents had access to NHS services, nor how the service is funded in toto. The basis of health care provision in the UK since 1946 has been for universal access, largely free at the point of use. These services are principally funded through general taxation. The NHS encompasses primary and secondary care, community care and ambulance services. There are a number of 'grey areas', principally the interface with social services (which is part of local government), which has responsibility for 'social care', and dentistry, which ostensibly remains part of the NHS but is drifting towards private practice as large numbers of dentists are refusing to treat NHS cases, complaining that the level of remuneration is too low.

Whilst these 'anomalies' frustrate those seeking to present the NHS as a coherent, universal and logical set of services and give ammunition for those suspecting a programme of privatization by stealth, the fact remains that since its inception both Conservative and Labour governments have retained a public commitment to the principles of NHS provision.

If the Conservative government's reforms did not change the essentials of state provision, they certainly had an impact on the way services were delivered. Prior to 1991 there was no formal distinction between purchasers and providers within the NHS. Health services were organized via geographically based capitation-funded health authorities typically comprising a number of acute hospitals and peripheral community services with primary care operating under parallel but administratively distinct bodies known as family health services authorities (FHSAs). The 1991 act created a formal purchaser–provider system whereby the health authorities relinquished control of hospitals and community services (which were organized as 'self-governing bodies' known as NHS trusts). Health authorities continued to receive capitation-based funding from government which it used to purchase services via 'contracts' or 'service agreements' from providers – thus the 'internal market' was created. FHSAs remained until April 1996 when a further act of parliament[9] led to the creation of unified authorities.

From the outset it was clear that a key challenge for government would be to strike the right balance between competition and regulation. In the first couple of years there was a particular emphasis on ensuring any change was gradual and controlled, with watchwords such as 'steady state' and 'smooth take-off' much in evidence. What all parties were 'taking off' to appeared to be a managed market, where the aim was to obtain the efficiencies of market systems (by creating incentives) whilst still regulating proceedings to prevent market failures.

As every government which has attempted this balancing act has found out, this is no easy task. The problem, simply put, is that central intervention threatens to weaken incentives and dilute market signals, rendering redundant the reform process itself. However, unregulated competition carries its own dangers, particularly in such an unusual 'market' as health care. It is highly prone to anticompetitive behaviour and 'market failure' may be considered socially unacceptable. The danger was always that the UK would end up with the worst of both worlds: 'a mixture of old style bureaucratic controls coupled with the additional transaction costs of the market and without the benefits of either approach'.[10]

There is little question that some five years into the reform process the Conservative government feels vulnerable on this issue. As far as the author is concerned, effective purchasing is dependent on at least three conditions being present:

- a reasonable degree of autonomy and/or a central mandate to take decisions on issues of clinical effectiveness, provider capacity and provision of services

- access to decent information concerning the quality and cost of services being purchased and the financial and human resources to make use of this

- a mechanism for understanding the services being purchased and establishing a reward system based on their value. It presupposes the existence of – but is greater than – a coherent set of contracting methodologies.

Health authorities were disadvantaged in all three areas from the beginning. The Achilles' heel of NHS commissioning is its dependence on political will to effect change. When this is lacking (which has been the norm beyond the 'steady state' years) health authorities in particular are effectively neutered.

The purchasing function had to be developed in the UK as there was little relevant experience of the necessary skills to be found within the NHS. Likewise, contracting, costing and information systems needed developing – in some cases from scratch. The relevance of this book is testimony to the work still required in these fields. It would not be stretching a set of similes too far to compare the learning curve to that encountered by would-be eastern bloc capitalists making the transition from the Soviet central planning system.

By contrast, the American health care system seems much better equipped by reference to these criteria (something of a paradox given the assessment earlier in this chapter that the NHS was better equipped to tackle the 'macro-issues' of health care). This is not to say that American health care companies are by definition effective purchasers nor that there is no room for improvement. However, health authorities continue to struggle to make significant progress in all three areas and there remains a significant body of opinion that sees contracting and health authorities as irrelevant 'on costs' to the NHS. Will[11] spoke for many when he wrote that 'The plain truth is that contracting is irrelevant to the healthcare that most patients receive'.

However, the government did not provide health authorities with a monopoly on purchasing, as *Working for Patients* established two models of purchasing – one centred on health authorities and the other on general practitioners (GPs). The latter, known as fundholding, is discussed in some detail in Chapter 4, but for the present it should be noted that this self-styled 'wild card' has been the subject of considerable controversy. Whatever its merits, it represents a policy development which threatens to bring the organizational structures of US style managed care and the NHS much closer together and, as will be explained, much of this is likely to survive a change of government (albeit renamed and repackaged for public consumption).

Figure 1.1 outlines the structure of NHS health care as of April 1996.

One of the most controversial features of fundholding has been its method of funding. Health authorities are funded through a capitation formula and are expected to purchase a comprehensive set of services

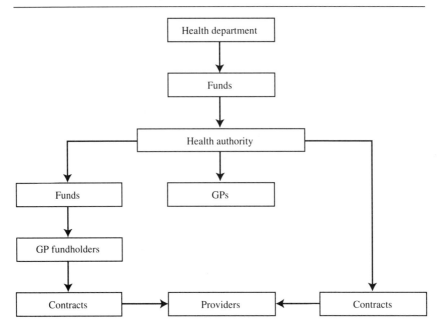

Figure 1.1: Structure of NHS health care as of April 1996.

from a population-based perspective. Fundholders' budgets are based on historical activity and represent a more limited list of services (principally of elective cases). The anomalies this creates are explored later, but for the present observations are limited to the fact that the fundholding initiative was based on the perceived advantages of establishing local, clinically informed decision making with direct financial advantages to clinicians for assuming responsibility for resources (and reducing overall expenditure). This idea has an international pedigree and developments in this field are keenly watched because the essential features, advantages and problems of such an initiative are relatively consistent between health systems.

Since its announcement in 1991 the government has worked to extend the scheme both in terms of numbers of GPs participating and what services it covers. The proportion of England's population covered by the scheme increased from 7% in 1991/2 to 40% in 1995/6.[12] In the UK overall, 16 737 GPs (51.62% of all GPs) were fundholders as of April 1996.[13]

Ministers have been keen to publicize what they see as the considerable success of fundholding. Ham and Shapiro[12] describe this official enthusiasm as 'treating it as the jewel in the crown of the NHS reforms'.

However, a review of fundholding by the Audit Commission[14] was less than complimentary about many aspects of the scheme's mechanism (inequitable funding formulae, high transition costs, etc.) and sceptical about its impact on purchasing. This has been seized upon by the scheme's many critics, including the Labour party.

The Labour party's policy on the two central tenets of Conservative health reform – the internal market and fundholding – is, on face value, simple. They have spent over half a decade attacking it as fundamentally misconceived. They are publicly committed (as far as the term has meaning for a party which has been in opposition since 1979 and has made many changes to its policies in that time) to abolishing both the internal market and fundholding. Yet when one examines Labour's proposed alternatives, it is less than clear to what degree these differ from Conservative policy – in substance if not in style.

The first point to make is that the confrontational nature of parliamentary politics tends to mask the significant areas of broad agreement between government and opposition on the NHS. Despite each party's systematic and ritualistic attacks on each other's policy, the substance of their antagonism is often more imagined than real. The same might be said for US Congress, where the Republicans spent a considerable amount of time and money demolishing the Clinton Health Plan, only to put forward a series of measures on Medicare (a federally funded insurance policy for US citizens aged 65 years and over) which to the outside observer looked suspiciously similar to that proposed by Democrats only two years previously. These proposals in turn have been the subject of sustained opposition by the Clinton administration!

Both in America and the UK the principal parties believe they have substantive philosophical differences in the way their respective health systems should be operated, but such claims often look less secure when subjected to a thorough analysis. Margaret Beckett, the shadow health secretary, reflected this (although there are doubts that she would readily accept the inference) when she said in 1995 that 'the Conservatives are divided on whether to accuse us of accepting what they have done or wanting to destroy it'.[15]

As noted, the key difference of opinion between Labour and Conservatives has been on the costs and benefits of the 'internal market' and fundholding. Labour's hostility to both can be summarized as regarding the former as having no role to play in health care, but merely introducing useless transaction costs – trusts, contracts, bureaucracy – and on the latter, that fundholding threatens the equity principle of the NHS and also has high transaction costs. Labour wrap their criticisms in a general 'bureau-scepticism'. Money for service development is to be found from cutting management and transaction costs as Harriet Harman (Beckett's successor) reaffirmed in a letter to the *Health Service Journal*:[16]

> Our pledge can be financed from redirecting resources within the health service because we are committed to reducing market-related transaction costs. There is clear evidence that there has been a substantial increase in spending on management and administration since the introduction of the internal market ... We will replace GP fundholding with GP commissioning. That will end one source of increased administration immediately ... We will end the annual contracting round and replace it with our longer term comprehensive healthcare agreements between planners and providers based on cooperation, not competition. The money released will be permanently transferred to reducing waiting lists on a recurrent basis.

Labour policy on the NHS might be summarized as follows:

- abolish the internal market but retain the purchaser–provider split. Replace contracts with 'strategic agreements' of a collaborative nature. Trusts will lose their self-governing status but retain responsibility for the day to day provision of care

- replace fundholding with GP commissioning (described by Klein[17] as 'a nebulous concept which may turn out to be a euphemism for collective fundholding')

- continue trying to reduce waiting lists

- fund developments by efficiency savings within the service

- place greater emphasis on pay within a national framework, put an end to compulsive competitive tendering, and place more emphasis on 'democratizing' the membership of health bodies

- give continued support for clinical effectiveness programmes, research and development (R & D), audit etc.

Despite the ideological breast-beating that has accompanied this, a highly plausible case can be made for considering that this amounts to little more than a renaming of the existing structure. Admittedly, on a continuum of cooperation–contestability–competition, Labour proposes to push the NHS towards the cooperation end whilst the Conservatives are thought to favour a competitive model but the substantive differences may be marginal.

First, both parties remain immune from financial logic. The initial reforms were sparked by a funding crisis. The reforms themselves took no note of the issue, and hence every year since then the media carry a plethora of stories on funding problems for authorities and trusts. Labour looks set to continue this tradition. This will seriously undermine any hope of creating collaborative relationships between purchasers and providers, there being nothing like substantial deficits to sour relations between organizations.

Second, any system which purports to be delivering efficient and effective services requires a demonstrable system for mediating the relationship between those things customers want and the services being delivered. For sensible decisions to be made it has to be known who is providing good quality, cost-effective care, and who is not. This, coupled with Labour's ostensible objective of providing greater accountability and the common need for cost control, naturally implies strong systems of management and an infrastructure currently being attacked as needless bureaucracy. The author is confident that practical reductions in this area will prove marginal, particularly when it becomes clear that this will only serve to undermine objectives which already have a reasonable degree of consensus – the need for R & D, promotion of clinical audit, and the drive for greater use of evidence-based practices and clinical effectiveness.

Third, Labour shares the cross-party obsession with waiting times, and as a result will probably continue to promote the Patient's Charter and league tables. These imply an infrastructure capable of:

- monitoring standards

- accounting for any expenditure earmarked to tackle charter objectives

- reporting waiting-lists and activity.

Finally, Labour accepts the value of GP participation in purchasing and will wish to retain and strengthen current involvement. There are legitimate concerns about high transaction costs, the sustainability of the current fundholding scheme (Chapter 4) and equity issues, but any likely alternatives will not be without their problems. Labour is keen to eliminate direct financial incentives from GP-based purchasing but its problem in essence is that if it removes too many incentives it is not clear on which basis doctors can be persuaded to participate in what is increasingly seen as a daunting set of responsibilities.

Furthermore, whilst a Labour government may be able to reduce costs through the economies offered by multipractice agreements (although this often occurs via fundholding agencies at present), it will need to provide both management and information support to GPs. The means and organizational structures for achieving this would look something like the HMOs examined in subsequent chapters.

At the time of writing a win for the Conservatives would constitute a major upset (based on opinion poll ratings for the two parties). The chances are that a victory for the Conservatives would only result in a small majority in the House of Commons, so it is considered likely that the Tories would be content to let the reforms continue to develop into a more contestable and visible market. Deffenbaugh[18] predicts that:

> Fundholding would become the norm and GPs would take the lead in purchasing healthcare ... GPs would develop further into community-based integrated providers of healthcare services, leading US style health maintenance organisations.

It is possible that a re-elected Conservative government could be more radical than its predecessors and push forward the separation of public sector purchasing from its provision, allowing the private sector to take over the running of increasing amounts of what is currently NHS operations. With the structure moving towards a mixed economy model, there might well be an attempt to define NHS 'core' services provision with vouchers or private insurance schemes being introduced for 'elective' health care. This is the thrust of Labour's briefing document Road to the Manifesto[19] which states:

> The future of the NHS under the Tories is clear. If the Tories are elected again, they will strip the NHS down to the basic emergency services. For everything else, people will have to pay.

The pace of change may depend on who occupies 10 Downing Street in the UK, and the White House in the USA, but the underlying dynamics of health care provision make a return to the 'good old days' unrealistic. Both countries' health care systems are set objectives at odds with the means available to them and both could usefully learn some lessons from the other in terms of the techniques and trade-offs on offer.

In the next chapter the focus is on understanding what comprises managed care in the USA. This will provide a foundation from which to explore possible UK applications.

2

Managed care: the basic models

When you've seen one HMO you've seen one HMO.

Anon.

There are many different types of managed care organization, although the foundations from which they operate begin within a number of common assumptions or observations concerning the delivery of modern health care. They might be summarized as follows:

- the methodology used to reimburse providers has a significant impact on the efficiency of medical practice patterns. Therefore it is a primary objective of managed care programmes to create meaningful incentives for providers to practise cost effectively

- the service needs of large population groups are essentially predictable. As a result a wide range of services can be provided at a predetermined premium through defining appropriate clinical practice criteria, enforcing their application through effective utilization controls, and eliminating inappropriate financial incentives

- effective health care is also cost-efficient health care. Within this, that it makes economic sense – as well as being better for the individual – to try and prevent illness. As a result managed care companies and particularly HMOs have a strong primary care focus (by US standards)

- there is an overmedicalization of the population which results both in inappropriate treatments being performed and an undue dependence on medical services. Managed care attempts to influence this through a mixture of patient education, empowerment, and the aforementioned use of financial incentives which are directed both at the physician and the patient

- physicians play a key role in the delivery of services and hence in the expenditure incurred. Unless means are devised to influence their delivery of services the organization's financial viability is compromised

- a company cannot be successful unless it has a certain critical mass of financial, information and management resources.

All of the above could reasonably be described as characteristics of – or belief systems typically found within – NHS health authorities. Moreover, both organizations could fairly be described as having a concern for the health of their respective 'customer' base. Both wish to predict utilization of services, avoid unnecessary cost and inappropriate treatment, and promote the role of primary care and 'wellness' as a means of improving individuals' lifestyles as well as containing costs. As a result both countries' 'purchasers' are showing a particular interest in evidence-based treatment and the use of outcomes – and are likely to remain doing so whilst the efficacy of so much – relatively expensive – treatment remains unproven. In the USA, this initiative is being pioneered by the managed care movement.

As previously stated, the organizational structure of a managed care company will show many variations on a theme. There is no national model although certain shared characteristics (as above) are discernible. Managed care's roots lie in the insurance sector and in one sense HMOs and their derivatives are just the latest response to the perennial problem of how to provide affordable coverage and make a 'profit'. They have grown (in part) from traditional indemnity insurance companies' failure to constrain costs, and the propensity of health care providers to subject the population to medical practice variation (MPV).

To just examine a staff model (HMO, for example) would fail to illustrate the somewhat Byzantine complexity of the managed care product and organizations typically seen in the USA. Most of the models described in this book are drawn from the coverage options Sentara currently operates. This is by no means an exhaustive list. Moreover these 'models' are likely to change in response to market conditions. New coverage options may be added and existing products dropped. The organizational models which will be reviewed are:

- The HMO, of which one can find examples of:

  - staff models
  - individual or independent practice association (IPA) models
  - direct contract models

- The preferred provider organization (PPO).

The number of variations on a theme mirrors the predisposition of Americans to avoid plans which offer limited or no choice – of provider, benefits, hospital, etc. – and the varied ability and capacity of managed care companies to corral physicians into particular organizational and contractual relationships. HMOs are passed over in favour of more 'liberal' insurance schemes by many Americans because they believe managed care will restrict their choice, and this assumes an importance which may be lost on UK readers. Moreover, what by many in the UK would be regarded as a major advantage – uniformity of care – is likely to be viewed with suspicion by members of the American public, on the basis that it represents a means of driving the quality of health care downwards.

There is a continuous tension here between the desire to offer different models and products so as to satisfy and capture all potential members and the resulting dilution of managed care principles to the point where the term almost loses its meaning and plans cannot be effectively distinguished from conventional indemnity insurance products. It is common for a managed care company to put forward a portfolio of 'products', to a would-be customer (typically a company), hoping that in doing so they have the ability to satisfy the different (perceived) needs for coverage of the company chairman through to the shop-floor worker. Moreover, many employers will not consider a proposal unless such a portfolio is available – despite such variation increasing the costs of health care to all concerned.

Key characteristics

Before losing sight of the fundamentals of managed care via a plethora of brand names and abbreviations, its key characteristics and how it differs from ordinary health insurance are reviewed. Some of managed care's core operating assumptions have previously been outlined. The result should be an organization that aims to provide comprehensive health care to members in exchange for a regular (usually monthly) fee. Conceptually a managed care programme should be concerned not merely with providing care when a member becomes ill, but should be structured in a manner conducive to keeping the member healthy. In contrast, traditional insurance systems act simply as conduits between the providers of health care and the patient through the processing and payment of bills. However, this is a characterization of both organizations – managed care companies can compromise their preventative aims through their general cost-containment policies and contractual arrangements, whilst insurance companies are increasingly taking on board managed care philosophies and techniques.

Continuing the characterization, the 'typical' managed care member enjoys a 'complete' range of health care services within a defined network in return for a standardized fee. There will be few additional charges.

Traditional health insurance in contrast (which is still the predominant form of coverage in the USA) typically has a more restricted range of benefits, e.g. hospital only, which will leave a more significant amount to be paid by the patient, but allows much greater choice of provider and will not typically require either patient or doctor to undertake external authorization checks prior to a proposed treatment or procedure.

Transatlantic misconceptions

Two common misconceptions in the UK are that the premium (or cost to the member) for an HMO will be lower than that available via traditional health insurance and that employers naturally prefer to get their employees' health insurance from managed care companies.

In reality, a basic indemnity package (for a healthy individual) is likely to cost considerably less per month than an HMO premium. However, the two 'products' are not the same. Indemnity insurance will not be comprehensive, in either the services provided – for example, mammography examinations as part of well-women screening will probably not be covered – or the costs of care, typically through the application of deductibles, copayments and coinsurance (Table 2.1).

Table 2.1: Common insurance payment clauses

Deductibles	A fixed sum of money which the individual must pay each year for medical services before insurance coverage comes into effect. It operates in the same way as normal car or house insurance packages. For example, a deductible might run at $500 per year, so that the individual pays the first $500 of any medical bill before reimbursement begins.
Copayment	A copayment might be described as a mini-deductible, a small amount which the member pays towards each medical service, visit or charge, with the insurance company paying the remaining amount. For example, a flat rate $10 charge for each visit to the primary care physician or specialist, and $50 for emergency room and hospital treatment might be stipulated.
Coinsurance	This divides expenses proportionately between the member and the insurance company, say on an 80:20% basis. On a $10 000 bill the insurance company pays 80% ($8000) leaving the patient to pay the remaining 20% ($2000).

In most health insurance policies, the deductibles, copayments, and coinsurance come into effect together. The impact of this – particularly the coinsurance – is to make the financial impact of illness both unpredictable and, on occasion, very costly. For example, you go into hospital for an operation but this is the first medical service you have received for the year in question. Your insurance plan has a $200 deductible, a $50 copayment for the hospital visit, and a 20% coinsurance for all services. The charges are:

Room and nursing (5 days at $700 a day)	$3500
Tests	$ 800
Drugs	$ 300
Doctor's fee	$1600
Total	$6200

Clearly, insurance does not cover all of this $6200. There is the $200 deductible and $50 copayment. Of the balance ($5950) the coinsurance cost is $1180. In total the patient pays out $1430 and the insurance company $4770.

The above helps to explain why some Americans fall into debt when ill, even with insurance – the other principal reason being loss of earnings and loss of insurance cover when the nature of the illness results in a prolonged absence from work. It also helps explain why so many Americans have difficulty in understanding their own insurance policies (and the financial effects of illness).

Employers for their part will often fight shy of using managed care programmes due to a combination of cost ('Wouldn't it be cheaper if our employees just took out basic indemnity insurance?') and choice ('Our employees see their health insurance as part of their overall benefits package. They don't want restrictions on what doctors they can see, hospitals they can attend, and procedures that can be performed').

As a result, penetration of the employer market – although growing – remains incomplete, particularly in the case of small employers. Sales of managed care products to individuals remain insignificant in most of the USA.

Table 2.2 summarizes the key differences between traditional health insurance and managed care (particularly HMOs).

Once again, the information in Table 2.2 should be seen more as characterizing two poles of what is in reality a spectrum of products offered by traditional health insurers and managed care companies alike. In the case of managed care, the degree to which members and providers are locked into a regulated network depends in part on the 'maturity of the

Table 2.2: Comparison of insurance and managed care products

Traditional insurance

- free choice of doctors, hospitals, pharmacies etc.
- emphasis on payment of expenses associated with sickness or injury only
- does not normally cover preventive health care
- no geographic limits to coverage
- member's place of residence may be anywhere
- payment to provider and/or reimbursement to member based on filing claim forms
- insurer has no direct involvement in the delivery of care. It is a reimburser of eligible expenses.

Managed care

- choice limited to participating doctors, hospitals, pharmacies etc.
- emphasis placed on preventive health care
- routine preventive health care covered, e.g. eye examinations, immunizations, annual physical check-ups
- designated service area defined by size of participating network. Non-emergency care typically provided by one practice
- a member's place of residence must be within the organization's service area
- claim forms not normally required
- close involvement in the actual delivery of care, i.e. precertification, use of protocols, advance approval requirement for out-of-network referrals
- expenses more predictable due to limited use of copayment clause.

market': a phrase which is meant to convey the fact that the penetration of managed care – both in terms of members and on provider behaviour – is uneven across the USA. In certain parts (such as California), managed care is the predominant method by which citizens receive their health care. In other states or areas, penetration may be all but non-existent.

Sentara is one of the leading edge managed care companies on the East Coast, but traditional methods of both obtaining and providing health care predominate in the area they serve. In 1995 only 16% of the population had managed care membership. The West Coast is generally thought to be some years ahead – Californian HMOs in particular are often called the crash-test dummies of managed health care! Health care products, relationships and contracting methods are therefore in a state of continuous transition.

The typical American health care company recognizes the inevitability of change – even welcoming it for the new opportunities it brings. There is a willingness to experiment and where necessary to cut one's losses and try something new when things do not work out to plan, or circumstances change. These are character traits all too often lacking within the NHS. However, that such variation can also create a menagerie of products and relationships is perhaps best illustrated by the description of managed care models and Sentara products, examined below and in the next chapter.

Definitions

Health maintenance organizations are organized health care systems that are responsible for both the financing and delivery of a broad range of health services to an enrolled population for a prepaid fixed fee. An HMO therefore performs both health insurer and health care delivery functions (although it does not necessarily directly employ the service providers but rather ensures services through a series of contractual relationships). Set out below are the most common models of HMO: staff, independent practice association (IPA) and direct contract. The model selected depends on how the HMO decides (or is forced) to relate to its participating physicians. Unfortunately for those seeking simplicity, the managed care industry can give many examples of a single HMO utilizing more than one set of relationships in order to deal with different groups of physicians!

A staff model HMO has physicians as direct employees of the company. These doctors are typically paid on a salary basis and may also receive bonus/incentive payments based on their performance. These would normally be the tightest organizational models in managed care. Typically the physicians are set up in large clinic-like facilities which can also operate as 'urgent care' (minor casualty) centres. Often the doctors only see patients belonging to the HMO whilst the members cannot go 'out of network' – see non-staff physicians – without losing coverage.

This allows the greatest degree of control over utilization, costs and the practice patterns of the clinical staff. Offsetting these advantages may be member concerns over the limited provider network, the costs of operating a salaried physician workforce and their motivation, and the high cost of building expensive care facilities.

The most common model sees the HMO contracting with an IPA. These associations of individual, independent physicians or groups of doctors in a practice have been formed for the express purpose of contracting with one or more managed health care companies. The physicians are members of an IPA which has a separate legal identity; but they remain individual practitioners, retaining their offices and identities. Many IPA physicians continue to see a sizable number of non-HMO patients, and for these doctors IPA-directed patients will make up only a minority of their list – and hence income. This makes the IPA a heterogeneous community, which can lead to problems with physician compliance and commitment – particularly when the HMO's members make up only a small percentage of a primary care physician or specialist's caseload. Essentially this describes the tension between the desire to have a large, multispecialty network which is more attractive to members, and the greater control that a smaller selective network brings.

IPAs, like much else in US health care, come in various forms. One type of IPA might have been set up by local physicians and operate strongly as an independent entity. It may well contract with more than one HMO on a non-exclusive basis. This type of IPA might contain many of the functions found in a managed care company – medical care management, credentialling, reporting, etc. In other cases, a particular HMO may work in close conjunction with a particular IPA – setting it up and recruiting participating physicians to it. Typically the HMO has an exclusive contract with the IPA and provides a considerable amount of administrative, financial and medical management support. This characterizes the relationship between Sentara's Alternative Delivery System (its managed care division) and the IPA of South-eastern Virginia. Such can be the symbiotic nature of the relationship between HMOs and IPAs that on occasion it is difficult to see where one starts and the other ends.

IPAs can serve several important functions for managed care companies. First, they provide a mechanism for transferring risk through the payment of a capitated amount to the IPA which then assumes the responsibility for paying its physician members. Second, they help the HMO build up a broad network of participating physicians. Third, the IPA provides a vehicle for peer review, quality assurance, education etc., on behalf of the managed care company. In short it assumes the role of middle-man to a professional constituency which typically dislikes the idea of direct employment or dealings with HMOs.

There are four major disadvantages of IPAs from an HMO's standpoint. First, the IPA itself creates an organized forum for physicians to negotiate as a pressure group with the HMO. Second, as already noted, their loose structure can make utilization management and general governance problematic. Third, the role of middle-man may reduce profits and influence. Fourth, where there is a symbiotic relationship with an HMO it can make the latter vulnerable to any adverse financial performance of the former: i.e. if the IPA makes a loss the HMO may feel it has little choice but to provide financial assistance as the alternative is the dissolution of its organized network. This is why, if HMOs were given a free hand, many would prefer to enter into a direct contract relationship with physicians.

In the direct contract model, an HMO contracts directly with individual physicians and practices to provide services to its members. It will attempt to recruit a broad network and is likely to try and get contracted physicians to accept capitation so as to limit its own risk (as there is no IPA to assume financial risk). With no organized body to interface with physicians – as there is with the IPA – the advantages and disadvantages noted in the IPA model are effectively reversed.

Preferred provider organizations are a common form of managed care where members have the choice of using either in- or out-of-network physicians and hospitals. Members are offered financial incentives to use in-network providers as a way of attempting steerage. In Sentara's series of coverage options it distinguishes between a 'point of service plan', which retains a primary care physician (PCP) as a gatekeeper but allows the member to go outside the network at an additional cost, and its 'pure' PPO product which has no gatekeeper function. Both the providers who participate in a PPO arrangement, and the members who buy this kind of plan, do so because of their relative freedom. For providers this normally translates into some form of fee-for-service reimbursement and total freedom to see other insurers' patients. These much looser forms of managed care (particularly the latter) are reportedly the fastest-growing components of the managed care continuum. A PPO's resemblance to traditional indemnity insurance is such that part of the portfolio of companies like Sentara that are offering a PPO option becomes all but indistinguishable from mainstream insurance products.

Tables 2.3 and 2.4 show the current range of Sentara's health coverage options (as of December 1995), which help to illustrate the essential models of managed care a potential member might opt to join.

This chapter ought to have conveyed some idea of the diversity of US health care without losing the reader in a sea of acronyms and organizational forms. It is important to try and convey this complex, rapidly evolving environment so as to make sense of the reimbursement models, structures and costs one sees in US health care in general and managed care in particular. This also sets the scene for the detailed examination of a managed care company contained in the next chapter.

Table 2.3: Sentara's group health coverage options (as of January 1996)

	Sentara Health Plan (SHP)	Optima Health Plan (OHP)	Sentara Point of Service (POS) – underwritten by Sentara Health Insurance Company	Sentara Preferred Provider Organization (PPO) – underwritten by Sentara Health Insurance Company	Sentara Out-of-Area Plan – underwritten by Sentara Health Insurance Company
Product/definition	An HMO which provides a range of health care services including primary and preventive care to employees of small and large Hampton Roads businesses and municipalities	An HMO which provides a range of health care services including primary and preventive care to employees of small and large Hampton Roads businesses and municipalities	A managed care plan that offers Hampton Roads employees the flexibility to use either HMO or traditional indemnity coverage each time they receive care	An indemnity plan that offers Hampton Roads employees traditional indemnity coverage with enhanced managed care services, such as preventive care	A traditional indemnity plan for employers whose employees live out of the Hampton Roads area
Description	A mixed-model health plan in which primary care is accessed through a network of physicians employed by the plan as well private practice physicians who contract with the plan. Members choose a	An independent practice model health plan in which primary care is accessed through a network of private practice physicians who contract with the plan. Members choose a PCP who guides their	A health plan in which care is accessed through PCP for lower costs (HMO coverage) or member may choose to use other providers (without PCP referral) for care at higher costs (indemnity coverage)	A health plan in which care is accessed through in-network physicians and hospitals for lower costs or member may choose to use out-of-network providers for care at higher costs. No PCP is necessary	Traditional indemnity plan that allows the most freedom of choice of providers while offering managed care components such as precertification for hospitalization and outpatient surgery, and medical care

Table 2.3: *Continued*

	Sentara Health Plan (SHP)	Optima Health Plan (OHP)	Sentara Point of Service (POS) – underwritten by Sentara Health Insurance Company	Sentara Preferred Provider Organization (PPO) – underwritten by Sentara Health Insurance Company	Sentara Out-of-Area Plan – underwritten by Sentara Health Insurance Company
	PCP who guides their individual care, and refers to specific specialists when appropriate	individual care, and refers to specialists when appropriate			management programmes
How it works	Members choose PCP who guides their individual care	Members choose PCP who guides their individual care	Members choose PCP who guides their individual care	Members may choose in-network or out-of-network providers. (Preventive services only covered if in-network)	Members may choose any provider
	PCP refers to a limited specialist network when needed	PCP refers to a larger specialist network when needed	PCP refers to specialists when needed or member self-refers for indemnity coverage	Member self-refers	Member self-refers
	Copays for services	Copays for services	Copays for services when using network	Copays or deductible/coinsurance for services when using network	

Table 2.3: *Continued*

	Sentara Health Plan (SHP)	Optima Health Plan (OHP)	Sentara Point of Service (POS) – underwritten by Sentara Health Insurance Company	Sentara Preferred Provider Organization (PPO) – underwritten by Sentara Health Insurance Company	Sentara Out-of-Area Plan – underwritten by Sentara Health Insurance Company
	No deductible/no claims to file	No deductible/no claims to file	Members pay deductible/coinsurance and file claims when using indemnity coverage. (Members responsible for pre-authorization for certain services when using indemnity)	Members pay deductible/coinsurance and file claims when going out of network. (Members responsible for pre-authorization for certain services when using indemnity)	Members pay deductible/file claims with a coinsurance arrangement. (Members responsible for pre-authorization for certain services when using indemnity)
Benefits coverage	Maximum coverage offered by plan		Benefit coverage decreases →		Minimum coverage offered by plan
Premium costs	Lower premium rates		Premium rates rise →		Higher premium rates
Provider network	Limited provider network		Provider choice increases →		Unlimited provider network
Funding options	All plans can be offered under a fully- or self-insured basis				

Table 2.4: Sentara's individual health coverage options

	Sentara Medicare Choice (SMC) – underwritten by Sentara Health Plan	Sentara Family Care (SFC) – underwritten by Optima Health Plan	Sentara Individual Health Plan – underwritten by Sentara Health Insurance Company
Product/ definition	An HMO alternative to Medicare which offers all the benefits of Medicare and a supplemental plan, as well as additional preventive care benefits, specially designed to meet the health care needs of seniors in Hampton Roads	An HMO alternative to Medicaid/ Medallion which places an emphasis on primary and preventive care, as well as health education, and provides 100% coverage at no cost	A point-of-service plan for individuals currently uninsured or otherwise not eligible to receive health benefits through their employer. This single plan* combines a more economical managed care schedule of benefits that has a limited provider network and a traditional indemnity plan that offers the freedom to see the provider of choice
Description	No claims to file No deductibles Optimal prescription drug programme No pre-existing conditions Preventive dental, vision, hearing and physical exams Regular health screenings and education Membership in Sentara Select Plus	• Preventive care (well-baby check-ups, physicals) • Prescription drugs • Selected non-prescription medications • Inpatient and outpatient hospital stays covered at 100% • Preventive dental, vision, hearing and physical exams • Regular health screenings and education	When using your managed care benefits: • Inpatient/outpatient hospital stays covered at 100% after $150 copay • Preventive care coverage • No claims to file • Prescription drug coverage† • Specialist care with referral When using your indemnity benefits: • Inpatient/outpatient hospital stays covered at 75% after deductible • Freedom to choose any provider • No referrals needed

Table 2.4: *Continued*

	Sentara Medicare Choice (SMC) – underwritten by Sentara Health Plan	Sentara Family Care (SFC) – underwritten by Optima Health Plan	Sentara Individual Health Plan – underwritten by Sentara Health Insurance Company
How it works	Low monthly premium. Copay – no deductible. Members choose PCP who guides their individual care	No premiums. No copays. Members choose PCP who guides their individual care	Managed care side: • Monthly premium • Copay – no deductible • Members choose PCP who guides their individual care Indemnity side: • Monthly premium • Deductibles and percentage of charges • Member responsible for precertifications
Premium costs	$35 per month $61 with pharmacy coverage	• No cost	• Premiums based on member health assessment**

* Available the first quarter of 1996, Sentara Health Plan will introduce a managed care plan for individuals without a point-of-service option.
** The individual product is underwritten on an accept/decline basis.
† Prescription drug coverage is with $10 copay or 30% of cost of prescription (whichever is greater) at participating pharmacy to an annual limit of $3000.

3

The anatomy of a managed care company

You can't buy widgets for a dollar, sell them for 80 cents, and make it up on volume.

Anon.

This chapter has two objectives. The first is to present a breakdown of the operations contained in a 'typical' managed care company (as far as such a specimen can be said to exist). In doing so, it serves to highlight the complexity of operating in the US health care market and helps to explain the unusually high administrative costs. The second objective is to give a pointer to some functions NHS authorities do not undertake very well at present, and highlight those additional tasks that would have to be undertaken should the UK turn to an increasing reliance on private health insurance yet retain a core of publicly funded services and/or continue to devolve purchasing to practice level.

Sentara alternative delivery system (ADS) – an overview

The alternative delivery system (ADS) employs approximately 400 whole-time equivalents (WTEs) and as of 1 December 1995 had over 210 000 members (excluding mental health) and revenues in the region of $220m. This makes for a ratio of just under two WTEs per 1000 members (about the average for the industry as far as the author was able to ascertain) and administration costs of about 15%. By contrast the author's current employer, Dyfed Powys Health Authority, has been set a target establishment of just 120 WTEs and an administrative budget of just 1% of its revenue allocation. With a residential population of around 500 000 Dyfed Powys Health Authority would employ some 1000 staff by US benchmarks, whilst the management target set for the five health authorities in Wales (which serve a population of 2.9 million) is just 650 WTEs in total.[20] However, the comparison is not entirely fair given that we are not comparing apples with apples as will be demonstrated below.

Characterizing ADS as a single company is somewhat misleading. It comprises five interrelated 'plans', two of which have a distinct legal status, separate accounts etc., and all of which are separately registered with the regulators. Each plan is attempting to satisfy a component of the local managed care market, and all are interlinked in terms of the support systems and staff operating at ADS. The reader need not be detained by the background to this complex organizational relationship except to note that it is a characteristic of US health care that if something can be complicated, fragmented, or otherwise given a distinct legal and regulatory status – it will be.

ADS's particular form mirrors this, but it is also the result of accident and history as well as design. At the time of writing it had both profit and not-for-profit examples, federally regulated and non-regulated plans, and staff and IPA models; some were wholly-owned entities, but one was 20% owned by another company! It is likely (although not certain) that over time these will be rationalized into a single HMO. For the present, it should be noted that such organizational complexity – whatever its regulatory and tax advantages – comes with absolute and relative costs, in increased administrative complexity, and the time spent by management in sorting through such a complex structure's affairs. Ultimately, these costs are passed on to the individual, company or government agency purchasing health care.

Membership and revenues for each of the five 'plans' vary significantly, representing, amongst other things, the maturity of the particular 'market' in terms of the acceptability of managed care to potential members (for example Medicare beneficiaries in the local area had largely yet to be persuaded of the benefits of joining an HMO), the adequacy and popularity of the provider network, the breadth of each plan's benefits, and its relative competitiveness when compared with other companies' products.

Summary of health plans

The Optima Health Plan has a membership of around 75 500, and an annual revenue of around $105 000 000. It is a not-for-profit HMO which at the time of writing was 20% owned by a third party. The physician network is provided by the IPA of South-eastern Virginia which has an exclusive contract with Sentara. Its membership is comprised almost entirely of commercial groups (firms).

The Optima Health Plan (Medicaid) has a membership of around 47 500 and an annual revenue of around $66 500 000. This is a more recent plan designed specifically for the Medicaid population. It has enjoyed rapid growth as the state has effectively subcontracted the management of the Medicaid programme to managed care companies who assume full risk for members' utilization of services on a capitated rate which is 95% or less than the state's historical payment for Medicaid recipients under the traditional fee-for-service system. The arrangement thus guarantees a reduction of state expenditure assuming a stable Medicaid population. Plans such as Optima's hope to make money through the use of effective utilization review, quality assurance and the primary care network. The latter has a particular importance in this type of population as typically 70% are beneficiaries of aid to families with dependent children (AFDC) and related programmes (in effect single/teenage parents) and traditionally are very high utilizers of emergency rooms and secondary care in general. Notwithstanding an HMO's ability to reduce hospitalizations via the above, it should be clear that assuming full risk for utilization makes Medicaid contracting a considerable challenge both organizationally and financially. The principal concern of patient interest groups and professional lobbies is that HMOs will only be able to make a profit by denying appropriate care.

The Sentara Health Plan (SHP) has a membership of around 42 000 people and an annual revenue of around $64 000 000. This is a for-profit HMO wholly owned by Sentara. Its network of primary care physicians consists principally of 'salaried' doctors, the remainder coming from the IPA network previously noted. The major difference between those who choose SHP over Optima is that the former is a plan with tighter control and a more limited choice of physicians offered at a lower premium.

The Sentara Health Plan (Medicare) has a membership of around 3500 and an annual revenue of around $15 000 000. Like Medicaid, this SHP 'spin off' has been designed to penetrate the large Medicare market. Medicare members pay a premium (in 1995 it was $35 per month with an additional payment if the member wanted drugs coverage). Competition in the market may lead to the elimination of premium payments in the future (although an additional fee for drug coverage is likely to remain) to which is added a health care financing administration (HCFA) capitation payment to SHP. In return SHP assumes full risk for these patients. The advantage for the patient is that normally they would have to take out supplementary insurance to cover those expenses Medicare does not cover. In theory, for their SHP premium they get better coverage for the same or less money than they would pay out in supplemental insurance. As can be seen by the modest membership numbers, persuading this population of the benefits of managed care has not been easy. This has been put down to a number of factors, including:

- the limited network SHP has compared to the total physician community

- reluctance of the elderly to change physicians they may have been seeing for many years

- concerns over restrictions on choice

- concerns that managed care means less care, etc.

Moreover, assuming risk for an elderly membership can be as difficult a proposition as it sounds, to which can be added particular problems with adverse selection (see section in this chapter on underwriting, p. 47). In short, although the common UK view of American health care is that it is a continuous 'gravy train' of easy profits and inflated salaries, it is all too easy to lose significant sums of monies – particularly when trying to expand into new areas, market new 'products' and provide care to certain sections of the population.

The Sentara Health Insurance Company (SHIC) has a membership of around 10 000 and an annual revenue of around $7m. Sentara Health Insurance Company is ADS's operation for self-insured employer groups. In the previous plans an employer would pay monthly premiums to ADS who would then be at risk for utilization of services but would keep any gains made from underutilization. Self-insured groups typically buy access to ADS's network (services) but the employer group bears the financial risk for utilization of its members. They may decide just to buy network access, with the employer retaining responsibility for the adjudication and payment of claims, medical care management, etc., or they may contract with ADS to undertake a full range of managed care functions for it.

Why would an employer wish to expose itself to that kind of financial risk? There are two principal, interrelated reasons. First, the type of employer who might opt for self-funding would typically be a large firm, perhaps operating countrywide, which considers it has economies of scale on its side. Second, this is usually associated with a belief that its employees enjoy better than average health compared to the general risk pool. They consider that under normal contracting arrangements (i.e. the HMO taking the risk) their members will form part of a larger, less healthy pool and the premiums will be charged on the overall risk. In effect, the firm will be cross-subsidizing other firms' employees' health care costs (p. 47). This is a growth area of business within US health care as more firms switch to self-insurance, based on the advantages outlined above.

Sentara Mental Health Management (SMHM) has a membership of around 370 000 and an annual revenue of around $5m. Sentara Mental Health Management effectively operates as a separate business with its own chief executive, accounts, and administrative infrastructure – including medical care management and claims processing. Mental health services may be provided to a group as part of an overall package of benefits paid for in a single premium. In effect part of that premium is given out to SMHM to manage on a capitation basis. The ostensible reason for operating SMHM as a company within a company is concern for patient confidentiality, but there is also the view that this kind of specialized area is best served by a dedicated management, clinical and administrative staff (pp. 77–83 give a detailed examination of mental health management in the USA and UK).

Table 3.1 shows the ADS departmental breakdown for 1995/6.

Table **3.1:** ADS departmental breakdown (figures have been rounded up; revenue budget only)

ADS departmental breakdown	WTEs	Budget $	%
Claims/benefits and member services	165	5.7m	16
Finance	43	9.0m	25
Underwriting	11	750.0k	2
Provider relations	41	1.7m	3.2
Medical care management	41	2.7m	7.5
Marketing and sales	73	5.4m	15.6
Human resources	5	500.0k	9
Health education	3	535.0k	1.5
Management information systems	N/A	3.5m	9
Administration and office ops.	14	3.0m	8.8
Misc.	9	3.1m	2.4
Total	405 WTEs	35.9m	100

Claims/benefits and member services

This function might be described as the Cinderella service of managed care. It is likely to be the most undervalued set of operations in an organization of this type. Its relative lack of status in the pecking order of corporate life is probably explained by its being:

- a cost centre and not a direct revenue generator
- a safety net for the promises made by other departments, i.e. when provider relations set up a contract with a provider which is difficult to administer (say through 'carving out' certain procedures to be paid fee-for-service on a contract which is otherwise capitation-based), the administrative burden and the irate telephone calls typically fall upon the claims department
- an area consisting largely of routine operations
- a producer of data which others turn into management information.

It will be apparent when the department's responsibilities are described below that mismanagement of this function can have a host of negative implications – member and provider dissatisfaction, poor public relations, inaccurate claims liability estimates, substandard collection of due income – adding up to financial problems and a loss of members/providers. However, this area also remains a significant cost centre; in Sentara it constituted 16% ($5.6m) of total administrative costs and as a result it is an area where rationalizations need to occur if managed care is to make significant inroads into its high administrative overheads.

In Sentara the claims and benefits function has been organized into five dedicated service units (DSUs) under a vice-president of operations. They were organized so as to cover the whole area of claims, member enquiries and benefit functions for a discrete geographical area or employer groups. This was a recent innovation as previously administrative functions were split up into discrete areas – member services, claims etc. The principal problem with that approach is the lack of continuity in dealing with an enquiry or claim as it runs through the system and the resulting 'hand-offs' from one section to the next. The philosophy behind the DSU reorganization was to provide a more seamless service. The DSUs contain the typical range of duties found in Benefits administration. These include the following.

Member eligibility verification

Member eligibility verification is a very important function with a surprisingly large workload. Sentara's re-enrolment rate was high by US standards at 97% but member eligibility is a dynamic process. New groups are signed up, existing members change plans, add dependents, move jobs. Medicare and Medicaid enrollers have further complicated matters as they have a legal right to disenrol and re-enrol on a month-by-month basis (as opposed to the more usual annual option) – a classic example of government regulation adding cost to an already overadministered process. In the case of Medicaid, many individuals become eligible and ineligible for coverage through the year. In contrast, fluctuations in GP list sizes in the UK – and the administrative headaches they cause – seem modest.

Benefit interpretation

This sounds straightforward until it is noted that a typical managed care company will be offering multiple benefit packages to employer groups. ADS has over a thousand different benefit combinations as a direct result of it responding to the market – the difference between closing a sale to an employer group and losing the business may be agreeing to a 'special', for example adding breast augmentation to the list of standard benefits (this and other cosmetic procedures are usually excluded) for an increase in premium. Furthermore, HMO plans typically have a preset authorization process before a member can utilize services (for example the need to get your PCP's authorization before attending an emergency room – except in life-threatening situations). Failure to do so may well lead to the HMO refusing to pay the resulting bill. This type of claim needs to be adjudicated and may possibly be appealed by the member. As a result, benefit interpretation can be a labour-intensive process. (Appendix IV gives some examples of these benefit packages.)

Provider claims for service adjudication and payment

This can be even more labour-intensive than benefit interpretation due to the complexity of many provider contracts (as outlined above), and the varying eligibility for payment based on the member's benefit package and adherence to procedure. It may not be going too far to say the managed care industry is too innovative for its own good, in that there is a tendency to create new contractual and financial arrangements at a rate greater than the supporting administrative infrastructure can assimilate. This even has its own acronym, OWA, standing for 'other weird arrangement'!

Member reimbursement for services

Most (if not all) services to members will be free at the point of use (beyond copayment). However, on occasion members may have made a payment and will seek reimbursement for services which once again will require adjudication.

Authorization of services

Both providers and members make enquiries about whether a particular service is covered. For example the State of Virginia Medicaid programme which Sentara covers (p. 31) excludes any coverage for abortion under any circumstances. The company has to comply with this – essentially political – exclusion under the terms of the state licence despite the fact that Medicaid already has a very high enrolled population of teenage and single mothers on welfare! There is an element of duplication of this function with the medical care management department who are also likely to field this type of enquiry.

Capitation accounting and payment

Certain providers will be paid on a capitation basis. They continue to submit claims for these services so that a track of actual service usage can be made. Furthermore, many capitation contracts have 'carve out' clauses and stop-loss provisions for individual cases exceeding preset amounts (Chapter 4). The DSUs provide the raw financial and activity data for other departments (finance and provider relations) to report on and use.

Liability accrual estimation

Accurate estimation of how much expenditure is being accrued is clearly important to any business. The DSUs have a major role to play in this. Claims are the principal means by which a managed care company spends its income (unless all services are capitated) and there is the significant problem of estimating 'incurred but not reported' (IBNR) expenditure. This takes two principal forms – expenses which have been authorized but not paid (which the DSUs should have a handle on) and medical expenses which the company has no idea of yet! The importance of the IBNR issue is emphasized in texts as diverse as Kongstvedt[21] and Weiner and Ferris.[22]

Kongstvedt states that 'unexpected IBNR [expenditure has] torpedoed more managed care plans than any other cause', whilst Weiner and Ferris go further, describing IBNR as a 'major problem' and predicting that when the concept is applied to fundholding in the NHS:

> The effects of the IBNR problem will impact on those services that are debited from the GP's budget on a service specific basis (e.g. drugs and some hospital

care). In addition to implementing accounting and billing procedures that ensure that all claims are reported promptly, the budget holders must construct lag schedules. These schedules are based on their experience with the amount of lag time between the date an expense was incurred and when it was reported.

IBNR issues will become a more significant issue in the NHS, (1) as the scope of fundholding GP purchasing grows – particularly should emergency cases be included – and (2) as contract methodology becomes more refined and 'block' contracts disappear. Obviously health authorities have had (and will continue to have as long as they retain any direct purchasing role) a version of the IBNR issue.

One of the most worrying features of any uncertainty in forecasting future liabilities within the NHS is the inherently low margins for error built into the funding system. It would serve everyone better if there were more flexible funding arrangements tied to financial plans that call for rebalancing budgets over a defined time period which were then enforced (in a similar manner to a commercial refinancing or rescue package), rather than the current arrangement in which many institutions lurch from crisis to crisis with structural imbalances between their liabilities and income which are rarely publicly acknowledged. The result is often a series of continued 'fudges' through a stream of supposedly 'one-off' cash injections and bookkeeping adjustments. Hospitals and health authorities in this position (and they are numerous) tend to adopt an attitude that their initial allocation, plus whatever deficit financing is made available at the 11th hour, constitutes their actual budget. The result is a stream of largely ineffectual firefighting operations aimed at the symptoms, and not the causes, of the deficit. When this goes on for half a decade or more it stretches the English language to call this state of affairs a 'crisis', as this implies a relatively short-term, unforeseen event. In reality, the position these organizations find themselves in is usually both entirely predictable and recurrent! These behavioural characteristics are further explored in Chapter 7.

Coordination of benefits

Yet another function exclusive to the US system, ADS has a dedicated team working to maximize revenues from coordination of benefits. Essentially, the job is to ensure that payment is made only once, where a person holds more than one insurance policy, and to reclaim part or all of a payment made to a provider from another insurance company (where that party has primary responsibility for its members' costs). This is quite common in the USA. For example, a husband may have Blue Cross 'family' cover through his work place whilst his wife may have a coverage from an HMO through her employer. Amongst insurers there is a pre-established agreement on the order of which organization has primary responsibility for payment. Coordination of benefits essentially avoids fraud by ensuring persons are not reimbursed twice for the same medical service. Substantial sums are collected through this process; ADS's target was to collect in excess of $4 million in coordination of benefits (COB) income during 1995/6.

Provider relations

The primary role of the provider relations department is the negotiation of contracts with PCPs, specialists, hospitals, and other facilities required to deliver the range of services ADS has promised to deliver to members in their benefits packages. The role clearly has similar features to the purchasing function within the NHS and specimen contracts are provided in Appendices I–III to help illustrate the points of both convergence and divergence. Key issues in both contracts are underlined for ease of reference.

Much of the department's time is spent building and maintaining the network to support the company's membership base and benefits packages. Unlike the NHS, a stable provider network can never be taken for granted. For a managed care company to grow it has to add members. Over time, membership in a given geographical area and field (employer groups, Medicare, Medicaid, etc.) will stabilize (perhaps to saturation point) and new members in untouched areas must be attracted. These members will want access to local doctors and hospitals – the average American has a very low tolerance to inconvenience in terms of travel time etc., despite the nation's justified reputation for organizing its society around the motor car. Provider relations must ensure an appropriate network is established and contracts placed. This function has no parallel in the NHS but probably occurs in a more limited fashion in the UK's growing private sector.

The above is a complex process because:

- the market is very dynamic. A network may need to be created in a 'virgin territory' in a matter of weeks (for example through success in the Medicaid contracting initiative) or alternatively rationalized due to a loss of members to competitors

- relationships are affected by the ability of the company to steer patients to the provider in question, that provider's utilization and quality of service, member feedback, the level of reimbursement being proposed, etc.

- there is a rapid evolution of managed care contracting arrangements. In general there are three discernible trends; to get all providers – including hospitals – to share risk on utilization, promotion of the role of the PCP as 'gatekeeper', and to ensure all physicians have adequate incentives to manage 'downstream' costs (e.g. referral to hospitals, diagnostic centres and nursing homes).

The latter point touches upon one of the major differences in emphasis between a managed care company's approach to contracting and that of the typical NHS purchaser. The former effectively negotiates access contracts with providers. Volumes are discussed in broad terms to effect larger discounts but what is not being attempted is to set predetermined volume at specialty or procedural level as many NHS contracts do (Appendix III). The contracting team will probably undertake modelling exercises on projected volume based on historical utilization for internal planning purposes, but it is unlikely that they will approach a hospital to contract for specific volumes, e.g. 400 total hip replacements, 100 coronary artery bypass grafts, or even at a specialty-based level – 3000 general surgery cases. If it did the company would have previously identified the projected case mix of those 3000 cases. This highlights a feature of US contracting techniques – the break down of caseload so as to understand its composition (case mix) before its build up again to negotiate a capitation or broad access contract. This is yet to become a routine technique for NHS contractors (in part because of problems with obtaining and then analysing the required data).

More often the primary focus will be on negotiating an 'access contract' whereby a discounted rate per procedure is agreed but the volume left open. Alternatively, a capitation-type contract is signed which effectively sets the funding per month to the provider – either as a percentage in dollars in proportion to the HMO's total membership, or 'contact-based' (Chapter 4 also reviews reimbursement mechanisms in detail). The latter approach is becoming popular as managed care companies attempt to tie in all provider bodies into sharing risk on utilization costs.

The principal difficulty with applying this approach in the UK (which is not that different from the traditional block contract in philosophy) is the problem of waiting list management and the continued growth in emergency admissions. This is not really an issue in the USA, as the premiums set generally assume a higher rate of clinical intervention than is common in the UK. Insofar as rationing takes place, it occurs through:

- the premium rate set – in effect rationing by the amount each individual is willing and able to spend on health care

- the pre-authorization and utilization review process, with each benefit package setting out excluded treatments (Appendix III). The medical care management process – described in detail in Chapter 5 – is designed to screen out particularly questionable interventions. However the US generally has a higher propensity to undertake surgery so the tolerance thresholds are more liberal to begin with. For example Schwartz[23] demonstrated that in 1984 the US, in comparison with the UK:

  - undertook twice as many X-ray examinations per patient
  - had three times the rate of kidney dialysis treatment
  - had six times the CT scanning capacity
  - performed ten times the rate of coronary artery surgery

- the risk-sharing arrangements with providers. Part of the underlying logic of negotiations with providers is that for the insured population there is more clinical activity being undertaken at a greater cost than is medically necessary. Moreover, provider revenues are greater than that required to provide quality health care. As a result, both clinical activity and payments can reduce without detriment to members or waiting lists developing. As anyone who has tried to negotiate a reduction in contract sum commensurate with lower levels of clinical activity knows, this is easier said than done, as NHS providers typically operate with a fixed income sum in mind. Though increased volume can usually be purchased at marginal cost, proposals that volumes be decreased are typically met with the response: 'If you decrease the volume we will have to raise prices.'

What is interesting about this exchange is how different it is from the behaviour of firms in more competitive marketplaces. Faced with reduced volumes, the typical response of such a firm would be to reduce prices so as to increase demand and to look internally for cost reductions. Whilst it would be naïve to think that this is the response of US providers on every occasion there is a much greater likelihood of this happening than in the UK. Economists would recognize NHS provider behaviour as more in keeping with a supplier that considers itself to be in a monopolistic position, or simply immune from market forces.

In fairness to NHS providers they are unlikely to enjoy the kind of margins that many of their US counterparts have to play with. This is compounded by a considerable national reluctance to rationalize capital stock and reform staffing practices. (This is further examined in Chapter 8.) For the present we are left with the observation that a principal component in market operations seems to be largely missing in the current NHS. The NHS has adopted the language of a market but not its reality.

The principal difficulty for NHS purchasers and providers interested in establishing a risk-sharing arrangement based on some form of capitated 'block contract' is that with demand already so clearly exceeding supply, creating additional incentives to limit the amount and intensity of work done is likely to aggravate further the waiting list problem. As guarantees in the Patient's Charter have considerably reduced the room to manoeuvre on this traditional safety valve, the pressure on the 'partnership' may become too great. However, such an arrangement may still work if the following three conditions can be met:

- both parties have a clear understanding of the historical and the future case mix
- mature relationships exist between purchaser and provider
- the relationship is underpinned with a sound contract.

If either party has failed to do its preparatory homework they will soon regret it when the costs of the actual caseload become apparent. The lesson once again is that it is necessary to break caseload into its associated elements *before* a total funding package is negotiated.

It is important that mature relationships exist between purchaser and provider. The internal market concept has required everyone to adopt new working practices, techniques and attitudes. The creation of both NHS trusts and fundholders has profoundly changed the institutional structure of the NHS. Unsurprisingly, the opportunity was often taken locally to utilize new-found autonomy in settling old scores. At the same time there has been a 'business practice' learning curve, with the starting point for some being the values of 19th century robber barons – conflict, ruthlessness, and a capacity for taking advantage of any perceived weakness of the other party – based on the mistaken belief that this is how businesses operate. This oscillates with an ironic tendency towards seeking bureaucratic redress from the 'centre' when intimidation fails. Such is the price being paid for the ambiguity in creating a market that is not a market.

It goes without saying that this is not the atmosphere in which a risk-sharing contract can successfully operate. More mature relationships are necessary. GPs may find it easier to achieve such relationships, in part because they will be more directly impacted by any negative consequences for patient care, and have less to gain personally from playing to a wider audience. Where such mature business relationships are believed to exist (by either fundholder or health authority with a provider) a full risk-sharing arrangement would be a significant test of its strength.

Almost in contradiction to the previous point is the need to reinforce the working relationship with a sound contract. Contractual safeguards act as 'due diligence' in an uncertain world. What kind of contract terms should each party be looking for? It is recommended that the capitation payment or 'block contract' has at least one, and preferably a combination, of the following 'triggers':

- a target total 'case mix' weight (total cases multiplied by their respective case weights) with a tolerance of say 3% on each side of the target. If the actual total case weight – perhaps monitored on a quarterly basis – stays within 3% either side of the target then the payment level remains unaltered. If it either exceeds or dips below 3% an additional or reduced payment kicks in at a preset marginal rate

- a series of projected year-end waiting-list positions is agreed with variance beyond a set tolerance level resulting in either additional payments or a rebate. This might be combined with the previous clause so that additional payments are only made when both targets are achieved, i.e. the provider cannot claim payment for additional caseload if waiting-lists have not fallen to target. However nor can the purchaser claim a rebate for reduced activity if the waiting-lists have fallen to target

- there should be clear definitions of what constitutes a readmission, double billing, etc. It is recommended that readmissions do not count towards total caseload (in effect that they are not reimbursed) and if possible that the cost of referrals to other providers be taken from the total payment to the initiating hospital. The purpose of these clauses is to minimize the opportunity for 'churning' and general manipulation of activity to inflate volumes, and transfer costs to other parties who can then make their own claim on the purchaser.

The above clauses go some way to addressing the following concerns:

- for a provider the purchaser (or more particularly GPs) will take advantage of a contract with no volumes to refer excessive numbers of cases to the hospital both as emergencies and to the waiting-lists

- that should case mix-based caseload rise, there be a chance of adequate reimbursement.

For a purchaser the provider will not manipulate activity and case mix (do the easiest and hence cheapest elective cases, either leaving the most expensive cases on the waiting-list or referring them on to another hospital):

- that activity be 'churned', e.g. through readmissions, charging both for a procedure undertaken following an outpatient attendance as a day case and also charging for the outpatient procedure when the work could have been performed and recorded as a single event, deciding that all cases referred for an opinion be considered suitable for further intervention and hence get placed on a waiting-list, etc.

- that activity will simply exceed the capacity of the purchaser to pay for it. This is a key issue, as identified earlier in this chapter. If either the purchaser considers provider activity inadequate to get waiting-lists down to the desired level, or the provider believes the contract sum is insufficient to keep the organization viable, the relationship is likely to break down.

In conclusion it may be too early for the NHS to embark on the type of risk-sharing contracts increasingly being utilized by HMOs. However, for those parties who believe they are capable of operating a capitation-based contract and have the will to work together in tackling the above issues, they have the opportunity to achieve that much sought after goal in business – the win–win situation.

Credentialling

Credentialling is a function often performed by both hospitals and managed care companies although in theory an integrated health system (such as Sentara's) could – and should – undertake credentialling in one department. At the time of writing, the ADS component sat in provider relations but they were about to start just such a process of consolidation with the hospitals Sentara owned.

Credentialling is the process whereby you ensure doctors have the appropriate licences to practise, insurance, qualifications, postgraduate training etc. This is a more complex process than in the UK, partly because a doctor may have admitting rights to one facility but not another, but also because there is a greater emphasis on attainment of predetermined standards and attendance of training courses before (for example) a doctor is allowed to practise certain surgical techniques, such as minimal access surgery. The NHS could usefully employ a more rigorous monitoring process in these and related areas (such as malpractice and complaints history), although setting out minimum training and volume requirements for procedures implies a willingness on the part of the service to fund appropriate courses and study leave which may in reality be absent!

Medical care management

The role of this department is covered in depth in Chapter 7. For the present we should note that medical care management undertakes the pre-authorization and utilization review functions which lie at the heart of managed care's strategy for monitoring and controlling the patient care process. It is also worth noting that there are areas of overlapping responsibilities between this department, provider relations and the claims and benefits function as one or all may be involved in the adjudication of complex cases and their repercussions in terms of relationships with the member and provider(s). Rationalization of this process to avoid multiple departmental involvement and 'hand-offs' between personnel is a major objective in the drive for internal savings and increased efficiency. The importance of adequate investment in management information systems (MIS) becomes apparent with this type of issue as it is very important that the organization operates a system flexible enough for all parties to use so as to avoid multiple data entry of the same information (Chapter 7).

Human resources

The personnel function is one area that contains very similar functions to its NHS counterpart, with the obvious proviso that there are no national personnel policies or wage agreements.

Health education

This department also performs a similar role to its UK counterparts, although its emphasis is considerably less on liaison with other agencies (city councils, police, education, etc.) on health promotion issues and more on getting a direct message and services to members and staff. One feature of health education activity at Sentara worth particular note is the extensive programme of activities made available to the company's 10 000 plus staff when they join its Healthy Edge programme. The programme provides a series of free activities for employees aimed at promoting a healthy lifestyle. One of the most innovative features of Healthy Edge is that upon joining, and from subsequently participating in activities, an employee can earn 'flex dollars' which go towards paying for health benefits. Enrolling (which involves an initial health screening and feedback to establish a baseline) qualifies an employee for a $15 reduction. Participation in each event increases the total to $60 per annum. The following free activities were available: aerobics, managing menopause, arthritis aquatics, diabetes class, humour therapy/stress relief, 'flu vaccination, health screening, smoking cessation, eating for life, healthy heart, yoga, professional image, walking and cycling clubs, and participation in charity runs and walks.

The Healthy Edge programme could also be purchased by employer groups for specific targeting to their members.

If the NHS seriously wishes to promote health education it could do worse than start with its own workforce. A similar scheme could be introduced, even including the particular organization increasing individuals' salary in lieu of the aforementioned 'flex dollars'.

Marketing and sales

As US health care companies operate in a genuine market, the marketing and sales function is extremely important. Membership has to be grown and then retained. New plans have to be marketed. A company that expects the public to come to it – to be aware of the manifest superiority of its products over those of its competitors – is in for a rude shock. A sizable marketing and sales budget is therefore deemed a necessary expense, but it is yet one more feature of US health care that the UK would be well advised to avoid. Considerable sums are spent on 'branding' the company's image and products (a positive side-effect of this is that US health care really does concern itself with quality issues and customer feedback, as these are often major determinants of customer selection and retainment) through brochures, billboards and media advertising. Sales techniques include the use of telemarketing and door-to-door selling for defined markets such as Medicaid, free telephone services, and a regular sales force dealing principally with employer groups. As managed care starts to penetrate the individual insurance market it is likely that increasing use will be made of independent 'brokers' who will sell managed care cover alongside traditional indemnity health insurance. These same brokers also sell life, car and house insurance and this is mentioned because it helps to illustrate the American attitude to health care – that it is a commodity, and is thought of in the same terms as the desirability of obtaining adequate insurance cover for one's property.

At Sentara both strategy formulation and public relations fell broadly within the marketing arena. There really is no direct equivalent of the traditional planning function seen in health authorities and regions and the paucity of strategy documents would be disturbing to the average

NHS-trained manager. The following reasons might be offered for this different approach:

- the health market is moving so rapidly that anything other than a broad outline of a company's intentions would quickly be out of date

- there is an associated need for flexibility. Planning documents have a tendency to become anchors

- there are commercial confidentiality concerns

- there is no requirement to submit regular plans to government bodies or consult with the public

- consistency is not really important, whereas profitability is. Yesterday's smart investment is today's dog.

The different approaches to strategy formulation and implementation are also discussed in Chapter 8.

Administration and office operations

In addition to the normal range of staff found in the chief executive's or president's office are those personnel who deal with the state and federal regulatory agencies and act as the interface with the company's attorneys on legal issues. Managed care as part of the insurance industry is heavily regulated. The regulatory bodies are concerned to ensure that the company is fiscally sound, that benefits sold to the public are uniformly administered, and that plans are being operated in the manner in which their original licence was agreed. In addition, the HMO replacements for state and federal schemes such as Medicare and Medicaid have a regulatory framework that must be followed at all times, including when rate increases have to be filed, and the type of benefit packages that can be offered under the schemes. Each health plan and company form has to be separately licensed. Once again this is a set of functions which has no NHS equivalent. One point to note – woe betide any organization that fails to follow state and federal regulations. At a minimum substantial fines will follow, if not court action. The point is, this is not simply a bureaucratic process. The regulators have teeth and have a demonstrated capacity to use them.

Management information systems

This department develops and maintains the information technology (IT) environment that increasingly acts as the core of the managed care system. As HMOs are data intensive and information dependent entities, a well run, adequately resourced MIS infrastructure is vital to a company's operations and long-term viability. The MIS environment in US health care is discussed in greater detail in Chapter 7.

Finance

The department performs a similar role to its NHS counterparts although it might be distinguished by a more 'liberal' approach to financial management issues. By this is meant that the finance role per se in the USA is essentially indistinguishable from other management functions, in that the chief financial officer does not see his/her prime duty as telling the company what it cannot afford to do. Financial solvency is clearly a major issue but it is a shared responsibility – arguably of greatest concern to the president/chief executive officer – and although many accountants are by temperament fiscal conservatives their role in the company is not necessarily to promote a balanced budget. They are charged with providing accurate, timely and understandable financial information, reporting on trends and highlighting for the management team pertinent financial issues. At ADS the finance department was responsible for a wide range of information reporting – utlization, length of stay etc., as well as expenditure.

It should be noted that US managers and physicians are distinguished by their generally much greater knowledge and interest in financial issues than their NHS counterparts. This makes the accountants' job both easier and more difficult, as they do not have to devote so much energy being the organization's financial conscience but they are more likely to be challenged on any projections/reports that do not 'look right'.

Underwriting

The process of determining and adjusting premium rates is arguably the most important internal activity an HMO undertakes. If it sets the wrong rates – too high and it becomes uncompetitive, too low and revenues will not cover costs – it will lose money and may go out of business. It is also one of the most controversial aspects of managed care with detractors arguing that HMO pricing policies are inequitable, using selection bias (enrolling healthier, low-cost employees and rejecting those most in need of health care) and pre-existing condition exclusions to boost profits whilst failing to deliver on the promises of effective and cost-efficient health care.

Rate-setting clearly is an important function, within the context of US health care, but is any of this relevant to the UK? There is no equivalent requirement or department within the NHS, so at one level the answer is no – although it is an important process to study for anyone attempting to understand US health care. However, rate-setting employs some useful techniques which have a more general application. Rate-setting requires an ability to predict patient utilization patterns and their associated costs. It presupposes an understanding of the impact of demographics, and as the consequences of setting the wrong rate can be dire, it is approached with understandable thoroughness. These are useful skills in any health setting.

Understanding the rate-setting debate gives the reader a clear insight into one of the key battlegrounds of health care reform in the USA. Also, those proposing a greater role for private health insurance in the UK must be able to address the issues raised in this chapter. In this context it is worth remembering that competition engenders new types of problems as well as conferring benefits. These problems have been magnified in the USA due to its highly decentralized, individualistic and pluralistic character, but exist to some degree in all competitive models for health care.

The rate-setting process and its relevance to the UK

It is important to remember that traditionally most members of an HMO join through being an employee (or family member of an employee) of a firm which offers health coverage as a benefit. A very sizable portion of an HMO's book of business comes from employers, however, the amount of income from federal state agencies to Medicare/Medicaid is growing rapidly, with relatively little coming from people joining HMOs as private individuals. The inevitable result – unless external regulatory controls mandate otherwise – is a focus on the part of employer and HMO of the particulars of the membership pool under consideration. In other words, if the employer considers his workforce and dependants to be essentially healthier than the 'average' he/she will agitate for lower premiums. Under these circumstances, the typical employer will resist any attempt to cross-subsidize or contaminate his pool with other, less healthy or riskier (and therefore potentially more costly) groups. The same thought processes are essentially at work in the underwriting or rate-setting department of the HMO. Essentially, healthy groups are preferred. In an uncontrolled environment the paradoxical result is that those most in need of health care have the greatest problem in obtaining coverage. Health care in the USA is considered by many within it, to be that country's most heavily regulated industry. Even so, there are enough examples of this problem occurring to consider the US health care system hopelessly dysfunctional, if one of the judgements of a system of health care is its ability uniformly to deliver care to the sick. There is a lesson here: in the absence of regulatory structures which mandate selection of unhealthy individuals, insurance companies, hospitals and doctors will typically behave in line with their self-interest and cultivate the healthy. The observation assumes particular importance when fundholding is considered. US observers such as Weiner and Ferris[22] predicted that 'under budget holding … healthy patients needing fewer services become more appealing and sick patients less so'. They went on to predict that: 'if a payment does not adequately adjust for need, serious issues relating to equity and quality are raised'.

For Weiner and Ferris the only solution is an effective case-mix adjusted capitation system – a lower per capita payment would be associated with healthier than average persons and a larger payment with those with greater morbidity – but this author would go further and require regulatory oversight of fundholder behaviour to ensure there was no selection bias.

This issue is part of what for many is a central difficulty in the further development of finances to GPs – the fear that non-clinical, i.e. financial, considerations will increasingly play a role, thus subverting the doctor's position as the patient's advocate, and undermining the doctor/patient relationship.

Unfortunately for the advocates of fundholding, even the most cursory examination of the history of medicine produces numerous examples of the influence of reimbursement methodologies on clinical practice – often with perverse effects on optimal patient care. One could go so far as to say that the practice of medicine in the USA is dominated by these incentives and constitutes the underlying premise of the managed care initiative described in the book.

Bevan et al.[24] have termed this influence on clinical decisions 'distortion by commercial considerations', and the issue cannot be either simply ignored or swept aside by platitudinous assurances about the ethical character of Britain's medical profession. One of the reasons total capitation as a means of paying doctors is only being tentatively introduced in the USA is the concern that certain doctors will provide suboptimal care to preserve their incomes through non-treatment (the opposite effect of the most common concern in a fee-for-service system).

In fact, the quadruple safeguards of medical care management, the regulatory infrastructure, consumers' propensity to switch providers and the fear of litigation probably make this less of a concern than it should be in the UK – where none of those factors exist in abundance. This would particularly be the case if GPs' personal incomes are influenced by their fundholding performance.

To the author the answer lies in first acknowledging the potential for abuse and explicitly weighing up the pros and cons of reform, and second to minimize such a potential by the strengthening of certain safeguards and the creation of others.

Health authorities will need to have their supervisory and monitoring role explicitly set out but, in addition, this is an area that community health councils (consumer watchdogs) should be looking to cover. However, the ultimate regulation and supervision of all services should lie with a national regulatory body – an 'OfHealth' – which should either set up as a new entity, or act as an extension of the existing health commissioner's role.

As previously noted, one area that will require particular attention – if the UK is to avoid one of the most undesirable features of the US system, adverse selection – will be the means by which a GP selects patients to join – and remove from – their list. A means will need to be found to ensure that doctors have no financial incentive to refuse to accept on to, or remove patients from, a list. The underlying premise should be that this should be an infrequent, auditable event in any case.

The recommendation that an overseeing regulatory body is introduced along the lines of Ofgas, Ofwat, and Oftel is not made lightly, and in the full knowledge that such agencies have a chequered reputation for effectiveness. The question as to whether an independent regulatory agency should be created for the NHS was recently explored in a leading article in the *British Medical Journal*[25] and also in the *British Journal of Healthcare Management.*[26] Without repeating the arguments in these articles in full, their simple answer was 'yes', because the market for health care is simply too far distorted from that described by classical economists to allow it to go unregulated. Local monopolies and uncompetitive practices abound, 'customers' have imperfect knowledge and suffer from the fact that there is an inherently poor principle of substitution in health. As one correspondent to the author has aptly put it:[27]

If I find myself dissatisfied after trying cornflakes, I can always turn to muesli next time I visit the supermarket. On the other hand, if my wife has inadequate treatment for breast cancer, and suffers from a recurrence, no appeal to substitutes is likely to be helpful.

The need for an independent body (whether this means extending the powers of existing independent agencies or the creation of a new entity is a second-order question) is paramount. Neither health authorities nor the NHS executive can be expected to do the job adequately. In the final analysis they will be unable to separate market management tasks from their many other roles and objectives. NHS management has been shown to be particularly weak in expressing a distinct professional viewpoint detached from government or civil service.

Another reason for regulation is that health markets (of themselves) are not particularly good at providing incentives for efficiency. Producing the desired results will require intelligence, determination and an unwavering desire to stamp out practices which are not in the best interests of the patient. Fundholding (and the internal market) may make doctors more sensitive to consumers. However, this does not mean consumers should be satisfied with a current organizational mantra that amounts to little more than saying 'trust me, I'm a doctor'.

We need to distinguish between those elements of health care which are likely to operate within a market mechanism, e.g. cataract operations, hip replacements and minor dermatological procedures, and those which require central direction and regulation. An external regulator would need to be aware of the impact on contestability of services of both geography and the relative costs of clinical interventions. The latter, in particular, is not a fixed entity as services may become more open to competitive influences either through technical innovation – the procedure in question becomes more easily undertaken – or the absolute level of funding available for the service in question increases. On the latter issue, the use of market forces to determine the appropriate price of, for example, a coronary artery bypass graft is considered more legitimate in the USA where the volume of operations and centres greatly outnumber their UK equivalent. Consequently, natural monopolies are common for this and many other types of clinical services within the NHS.

Finally, the current NHS experience of the internal market has led many to conclude that there can be no such thing as a 'market' in health care. This is incorrect as a blanket statement but has gained considerable currency, not least because such fashionable statements act as a form of mental shorthand for those who would rather not face up to complex issues.

The cut off point for determining 'floating' vs centrally determined price levels is necessarily subjective, but the author believes is best obtained through direct observation rather than recourse to any particular ideology. However levels of reimbursement are determined, they will require mediation through some form of contract currency and this in turn will need to be sophisticated enough to allow informed benchmarking to occur.

When we say the current state of affairs 'is not a market' we have to be careful to distinguish between those situations where a market does not exist – but could be created – and those where, to all effective purposes, it makes no sense to expect market mechanisms to work properly (i.e. if left alone they will produce undesirable results, however defined).

Technical issues in rate-setting

There are two questions which this section sets out to answer. One, what are the principal methods by which rates are set? Two, what are the major controversies in rate-setting?

Rate-setting methods

HMOs set rates within a regulatory framework, the most important being the restrictions imposed on federally regulated HMOs. These HMOs have to use a form of community rating.[28]

> Until the relatively recent flurry of development of nonqualified (mostly for-profit) plans offering experience-rated products, community rating was viewed by most HMO personnel as the only acceptable method for determining HMO premiums. However, the methods of implementing community rating have changed over time. Initially, community rating meant that there was only one premium based on the total experience of the whole community. More flexibility in community rating has been permitted through the 1981 HMO Act amendments, which allow community rating by class as an acceptable HMO rating method. Therefore, different premiums are often charged to different groups based on different mixes of classes of enrollees, and premiums are based on the experience of each class.

This is a complex subject and so a reasonable starting point is to examine each rate-setting method, beginning with community rating.

Setting premium rates based on community-rating principles (as originally set out in the 1973 HMO Act) involves in essence:

- determining premium rates projected on desired revenue requirements

- offering the same premium rates to all employers for the standard benefit package

- uniformly updating these rates.

The advocates of community rating argue that it is a simple system, allowing HMOs to charge affordable rates to all – including high-risk groups and individuals, by basing premiums on a broad-based community.

Limitations of community rating

The arguments for community rating appear convincing and indeed the claims for it have been demonstrated in areas where an individual HMO enjoys a high penetration rate and stable membership. However, in more competitive environments these advantages may lack substance. For example, community rating should promote a stable, predictable income flow. Yet should an HMO lose a sizable percentage of members to another competitor, then its revenues will be much lower than anticipated. Likewise, community rating is meant to promote premium-rate stability by preventing high levels of rate fluctuations. Should a competitor be able to attract a significant number of an HMO's low-cost members, the plan could find itself needing to raise rates very quickly.

Wrightson and William[28] highlight what they call 'the most common (and most dangerous) misconception (that) community rating eliminates the necessity for an extensive under-writing and rate-setting function. In a competitive environment, the competition is going to know the expected cost of all of its groups. By charging premiums that are related to the cost of each group, any significant changes in enrolment, because of massive enrolment or disenrolment of several groups, will result in similar changes in both premium income and benefit costs.'

Finally, as previously noted, there is employer resistance. Many employers believe their members will have a better-than-average claims experience and therefore cost less, and therefore gravitate towards experience-rated products.

Community rating by class

In 1981 amendments to the law regulating HMOs permitted a new form of rating – community rating by class (CRC). The principal differences are:

- instead of assuming that all members/groups are of equal risk, an HMO can identify a set of rating classes that correspond to different levels of risk and are based on identifiable characteristics of groups and enrolled members (age, sex, industry, family composition etc.)

- the HMO can establish rating factors for each risk class that take account of their particular utilization and cost patterns (e.g. males age 25 are only 60% as costly as the average male; policemen are 20% more costly than the average, after controlling for age, sex and other demographics etc.)

- these rating factors can be used to determine rates for different groups, so group-specific premiums are based on the characteristics planwide of that particular group's enrollees – but not on the particular cost experience/utilization of the group in question. Experience-rating remains prohibited.

The last point is best explained by use of an example. When the CRC rating factors are applied to a particular group, the premiums will reflect the planwide risk levels based on the class characteristics in the group. They do not reflect the actual utilization or cost experience of the specific enrollees of that group (as they would under an experience-rating system). So it is permissible to apply a different premium for firemen from office workers, but one cannot charge different premiums for, say, the fire department of Virginia Beach from the fire department of the City of Hampton.

The upshot of all the above is to give HMOs more flexibility in determining rates.

Experience-rating

The key features of experience-rating should be obvious from the foregoing. Private health insurance companies have used experience-rating as their primary method for determining group rates for decades. The general approach is to apply experience-rating on larger groups (over 250 members) and apply community rating on groups below this number. This is because of the high degree of random variation in health care costs for small groups year on year. Use of experience-rating implies the ability to monitor group-specific claims and make the appropriate underwriting decisions: a capability which insurance companies take for granted at their peril.

Controversies in rate-setting

Aside from the tensions between employers and HMOs on community rating there are other controversial issues which bear some examination. One of the most significant issues in both managed care and the US health care system in general is selection bias. One way to understand selection bias is to consider situations where it does not exist. For example, if people were randomly assigned to HMOs and other health plans, each company would have a distribution of individuals representative of the whole group. NHS health authorities with catchment populations drawn from large geographical areas may not satisfy all aspects of this theoretical model, but their 'membership' is as close to a random distribution as you are likely to get in the 'real world'.

Selection bias, in contrast, results in non-random selection of a plan so that the population characteristics of its 'members' are skewed. If subscribers representing higher than average risk choose the plan, then that plan is said to have experienced 'adverse selection': the health plan now has more than its fair share of high-cost enrollees.

From the perspective of an HMO, selection bias may be either 'favourable' or 'adverse'. It is favourable when lower than average expected risks enrol and adverse when higher than expected risks join.

Selection bias operates in the way individuals choose their levels of benefits. Overall, there is a tendency for persons who expect to be immediate or regular users of health services to choose the more expensive plans (which have higher premiums) but which provide the most extensive benefits. Conversely, healthy persons who do not expect to use services will tend to choose low-premium, low-benefit plans. This pattern of choice also applies to selected services. For example, if alternative health plans differ with respect to coverage of specific services (maternity care, mental health, substance abuse, vision care, prescription drugs) then it is to be expected that persons with a tendency to use these services will choose the plans with the best coverage despite the higher premiums.

A practical example of this behaviour, and its consequences in terms of adverse selection, can be given in the case of Sentara's Medicare product. As previously explained, the local Medicare population is wary of the perceived restrictions in managed care (supplementary insurance cover rests almost entirely with traditional Blue Cross/Blue Shield indemnity insurers). Sentara offered a basic product which traded choice for a good range of benefits, plus the option of a prescription drug benefit for an additional premium. With hindsight it is clear that the plan would invite adverse selection on two counts. The average 'healthy' Medicare recipient was not attracted to the limited network. The more unhealthy the potential enrollee the more attractive the product looked – people being willing to trade choice and travel time for large monetary savings. This was compounded by the drugs benefit option. Drugs are very expensive in the USA. Those enrollees with a significant propensity to run up expensive drug bills were attracted to the plan. The result is adverse selection and financial losses. Hence the twisted logic of the marketing staff's lament that 'we have to get healthier people to join the plan. Our problem is, we have too many sick people wanting healthcare.' That is the perversity of the American health care system in a nutshell!

HMOs and 'skimming'

'Skimming' is a term used for the deliberate attempt at enrolling the healthiest members of an employer's workforce, as their health care costs are likely to be lower than the community-rated premiums. Methods include:

- pricing practices designed to attract low-risk enrollees
- design of benefits to discourage sick or high-risk persons
- marketing/advertising directed specifically at low-risk enrollees
- encouraging high-risk persons to disenrol.

Some of these practices are legitimate attempts to enhance competitiveness and profitability. Others are unethical and border on being illegal. Employers sometimes accuse HMOs of profiteering via skimming practices – in other words their premiums fail to reflect their risk pool. It is obviously difficult to judge in relation to this, where the legitimate profit motive fundamental to capitalist endeavour ends and exploitative practices start.

One personal observation on the general topic of 'skimming' is that during the author's time in the USA he never saw a single advert for a health care company or service which pictured an ill-looking person! The subliminal messages appeared to be 'join our plan, come to our hospital etc. and stay healthy!'. Even the advertising specifically for Medicare products typically showed fit-looking retirees playing a round of golf. Consciously or otherwise such marketing appeared to the author to be promoting favourable selection.

Pre-existing conditions

One device used by traditional indemnity insurers to manage risk is the provision of pre-existing condition exclusions within their benefits coverage. This is commonly used by all insurers for individual and small-group coverage (often combined with a medical questionnaire/examination) and essentially states that the insurer is not liable to cover the costs for any condition that was diagnosed or being treated say three months prior to the person joining the plan. So, for example, if I have asthma and was being treated for this prior to joining the plan, I will be covered for this illness only if the expenses in question are incurred after the earlier of (1) 12 consecutive months of coverage, or (2) 90 consecutive days either prior to or following the effective date of coverage during which no treatment has been received for the condition in question. Not only is this yet another example of the problem the sick (particularly those with chronic illnesses) have in getting health cover in the USA, it is also time-consuming and expensive to administer.

Federal or state reform of this objectionable caveat would go a long way to improving access to insurance cover. The simplest way would be for the regulatory authorities to mandate all insurers to drop pre-existing condition clauses in their contracts. This would be painful for insurers but uniformity would mean that the pain would be equally distributed. This should also be accompanied by a mandate to all insurers to offer an insurance plan for individuals which had preset maximum (but not preset minimum) premiums based on some form of community rating by class (so as to ensure that insurers would not simply price themselves out of their obligation to offer coverage to all).

These two reforms would significantly improve access to health care and create a level playing field for all insurers. At the same time (by spreading high-risk patients across the industry) it would reduce insurers' concerns with adverse selection. As a by-product it should also cut down on administration costs. If the above were accompanied by caps on medical negligence awards and lawyers' fees, there would be a very significant reduction in costs without unduly impacting on America's market-driven system of health care. If anything, it would assist the market to operate more efficiently by eliminating opportunities for insurers to 'cherry pick' the population.

Copayments

The principal mechanisms by which copayments, deductibles, etc., operate have previously been outlined. These techniques can be used both to overcome selection bias and to control member utilization of services. With regard to selection bias the level of out-of-pocket expenses that employees and members must pay is a key factor. If the employer pays the entire premium, then employees and their dependants will be encouraged to enrol in plans with high benefits regardless of their health.

With regard to the UK the attractiveness of copayments (beyond its potential impact on the total finances available to the NHS) lies in the observation that there is abuse by some patients of current NHS services. The extent of this abuse (characterized particularly by frivolous use of emergency and GP services – including night visits – plus a widespread expectation of a drug prescription for self-limiting conditions and illness not amenable to drug therapies) is the subject of much debate and little research. It is also by its very nature politically controversial (not least because it strikes at the heart of a central tenet of the NHS – that it be free at the point of use).

However, would copayments work in the UK? The author believes the answer (with some reluctance) is no. There are four principal obstacles to the introduction and operation of copayments in the UK which together make up a formidable barrier to the copayment idea working successfully. They are:

- for copayments to be worth doing (income exceeding cost of operation and acting as a deterrent to abuse) the copayment has to be a reasonably significant sum (perhaps £15 a visit). Yet the very fact that it is a significant amount has two negative consequences:

  - it will put off some people from seeking treatment for themselves and family members who genuinely need it. This will have a negative impact on certain individual's health, and have possible public health consequences
  - the higher the level of charges the more discriminatory it will be on lower income and sicker members of society. Demand for basic health care provision is somewhat like that for food and other essential goods. That is, demand for these items is relatively inelastic regardless of personal circumstances. Moreover a £50 charge for being treated in the accident and emergency department has a lot less impact on an individual's disposable income if he or she earns £60 000 and not £16 000

- any amelioration of the above effects through exclusions and subsidies erodes the impact of copayments as follows:

  - the UK traditionally makes the following groups exempt from any of the NHS's current copayments (prescription drugs, dental charges) – children, pregnant women, the unemployed and other social security recipients, the disabled and the elderly. Whilst a legitimate case for exempting these groups from copayments can be made, every exclusion will reduce the rational for copayments as a whole – as anecdotal evidence points to some of these groups being the 'worst offenders' in terms of 'abuse' of services and they certainly represent amongst the heaviest users of health care
  - restricting the copayment levy to a subset of taxpayers reduces the financial case for copayments as a source of NHS funding

- an efficient and effective copayment process requires the NHS to have in place a sophisticated process for identification, billing and collection of debts. Although as a unitary entity with all citizens covered, this is a much easier organizational issue for providers compared to the USA (where hospitals and doctors typically have to deal with multiple plans each with its own copayment clause), would sufficient investment be made for this non-patient activity? Based on the evidence of current attitudes and investment, the answer is probably not

- there is unlikely to be sufficient political will to enforce such a payment system, and even if there were, copayments would likely become the NHS poll tax. Considerable, sustained hostility is inevitable, with many NHS staff and professional bodies likely to be in opposition. If the courts could not adequately enforce the collection of large sums of council tax* what chance would there be of collecting £15 copayment charges?

The final word might best be given over to a practical example of copayments in action. Whilst in America, the author was liable (over a 6-month period) for some $150 in copayments. This was in addition to monthly health insurance premiums. A total of $100 was spent on two visits to a hospital emergency room (ER) made with one of my daughters within a few days of each other. The rest was made up of $10 payments for 'routine' PCP appointments for my children – vaccinations, well-baby clinic, etc.

If copayments were introduced would there be tax reductions in compensation? Ill health is no respecter of class or income. Young children have a tendency to fall prey to bouts of illness requiring a spate of visits to the GP. As the bills add up over the year how popular would this innovation be, from London's stockbroker belt to the industrial north? So with some reluctance this US innovation cannot be endorsed. Unsatisfying though it may be, some abuse of the current system is probably a price worth paying for the many other strengths of the NHS.

Conclusion

In examining the operations of a managed care company many different areas of health care have been covered. A balanced picture of strengths and weaknesses has been given, and areas where reform is desirable have been highlighted.

---

* This refers to the difficulties the Conservative government had in enforcing changes it made to the basis on which local government revenues were raised. After a period of sustained civil disobedience, general public hostility to the scheme and non-payment, the 'poll tax' was abandoned in 1992.

In the next chapter there is a detailed examination of reimbursement systems and the issues that arise from them. In looking at various payment options and the wider issue of physician capitation, GP commissioning/ fundholding and the drive for further efficiencies, it would be wise to reflect periodically on the administrative structures available to support these initiatives.

4

Reimbursement mechanisms – paying doctors and hospitals

You can go on about physician education as long as you like, but if you really want to grab their attention you have to go for their pocketbooks.

IPA Board Member

This chapter starts with consideration of the role that reimbursement mechanisms play in determining and influencing provider behaviour within managed care programmes and the various options available to payers in setting up forms of payment. Some time is spent detailing these various approaches, before considering some key transatlantic issues, in particular capitation-based funding and the future of the NHS fundholding initiative/GP commissioning.

Whilst organizational structures and the nature of purchasers' relationships with providers may differ (sometimes quite dramatically), all managed care programmes utilize to some degree the following approaches:

- financial incentives that involve sharing risk with participating clinicians

- the use of approval mechanisms and financial incentives to influence patient and physician use of services.

Unlike in the UK, where there is considerable reticence about directly linking payments to clinicians with the costs of their method of clinical practice, it is seen as a reasonable goal of managed care that (all other things being equal) the payment system should reward the low-cost and penalize the high-cost physician. Arguably the introduction of fundholding has established such a link at practice level and therefore the US mindset is gaining ground. At the same time, consideration is being given to reform of the system of consultant merit awards and the introduction of performance-related pay for doctors. Under these circumstances the issue is more likely to be when the linkage will be made and to what degree, rather than whether it will occur. To US observers the surprise is that an explicit relationship does not already exist, given the pivotal role doctors play in the allocation of resources and the pressing need in the NHS to contain costs within set budgets.

Managed care contracts with clinicians will typically fall into one of a number of different payment systems, the basic variants of which are described below. Many of these contracts will in fact contain an amalgam of payment methods. They are:

- discounted fees
- capped fee schedule
- capped fee schedule with a withhold
- primary care capitation
- full capitation.

Each system results in progressively more risk being passed on to the provider. The more risk passed to the provider, the greater the potential gain to that doctor from reduced medical care usage and cost control. Conversely, the potential direct loss to the doctor's personal income due to excessive usage and cost is greater.

Discounted fees

This is a relatively straightforward payment method and is widely used by payers to both physicians and hospitals. In essence, providers (in this case physicians) agree to accept a percentage reduction on their charges/fees as payment in full, i.e. they cannot subsequently part bill the patient or some other party to supplement the payment from the HMO. Both physicians and hospitals typically discount their charges by various percentages depending on the payer. Large-volume purchasers and government bodies would normally get the largest discounts. From this it can be noted that US health care broadly maintains two market principles that the NHS has been instructed to ignore:

- the biggest customers typically get the best deals
- price equals what you can get the payer to agree to – not its cost.

Typically, with patients carrying individual insurance, and with out-of-area members of managed care companies, providers will attempt to bill at full charges. The variation in charges between payers provides HMOs with opportunities to lower prices, partly through cost-shifting to other payers who have less negotiating muscle. The purchasing power of large groups helps to explain the drive for new members which is a characteristic of most HMOs' strategies.

The implications for the NHS if it persists in operating what can only be described as a perverse economic environment for a system hoping to benefit from any form of 'internal market' is examined later in this chapter. Suffice to say that any government that establishes a set of relationships that typically gives the best deals to minority payers (e.g. fundholders) can expect some particularly abnormal results.

Returning to the use of discounted fee reimbursement for physicians in the USA, a problem lies in its use as a uniform payment method, i.e. if each physician experiences the same recovery from charges (say 80%) regardless of their charge level or number of services performed, there is no economic incentive to control charge increases or utilization. As a result, this type of reimbursement is fast losing popularity amongst payers in the USA.

Capped fee schedule

Here a maximum allowable fee (or fee cap) is determined for each procedure and the physician will be paid up to the maximum amount. The advantages of capped fee payments compared with discounted charges are twofold:

- they help limit the impact of any fee increases

- they are more equitable in that physicians with higher fees have to provide greater discounts than those with lower fees. Conceptually this is similar to the prospective payment systems for hospitals: diagnosis-related groups (DRGs), health-related groupings (HRGs) and chargeable procedures. However, since reimbursement is based on the number of services performed, and excessive hospital or referral services would result in no financial impact to the clinician, this system is not good at motivating physicians to limit services performed, use of hospitals, tests ordered, etc.

Capped fee schedule with a withhold

This approach is often employed by IPA model HMOs. A percentage of payment (typically 15–20%) is withheld from the physician and is only paid back if certain performance goals are met. These goals often relate to the use of referral and hospital services.

Although this payment method can create an incentive not to overuse services (on the basis that excessive utilization may reduce withhold returns), some physicians will not expect a withhold return (based on past experience), viewing it as a discount and increasing their use of services in order to increase compensation. There is also the problem of physicians manipulating the system to meet their particular targets. For instance, if a target is set on the amount of work undertaken by a PCP in his office and no relationship is made with his/her referrals to other bodies, inappropriate referrals 'downstream' to specialists and emergency rooms can occur.

This behaviour is also thought to occur within the NHS in at least five different ways:

- through division between primary and secondary care on responsibility for drugs expenditure. For example, hospitals sometimes prescribe drugs to patients of a duration and brand that minimize their drugs bill but increase the cost of the drugs bill to GPs (and ultimately the Exchequer), due to differential pricing of the drug charged to hospitals and the cost 'at the high street' retailer. This tension is likely to remain, as long as GPs and hospitals have their own drug budgets and distinct incentives to view the costs of health care as a series of isolated pockets

- the division of responsibilities between health and local authorities with the resulting 'grey' areas in community care and special education create similar cost-shifting opportunities and tensions between agencies. As with the aforementioned drugs issue this is always likely to occur when financial responsibility for the continuum of care sits with more than one agency

- the limited extent of chargeable procedures in fundholding provides opportunities for cost-shifting for those prepared to make the effort to do so – for example through reclassification and sending in cases as emergencies (which fall under the health authorities' funding umbrella)

- GPs have a set quota of minor surgical procedures they can perform themselves and receive reimbursement from the health authority under general medical services (a non-cash limited part of the health authority's budget). Once this quota is met new cases may be referred to the hospital (typically at a greater cost), with the cost met by the health authority from part of this cash-limited budget. This is another example of government regulation creating unnecessary costs, but a recently announced liberalization[29] of procedures which can be performed in a primary care setting may well reverse this process

- GPs have considerable latitude concerning whether to care for someone in the community or admit them to hospital. Until the advent of fund-holding there was no direct incentive to avoid making the most costly decision (and this remains the case for emergency admissions for all but the handful of 'total fundholding' pilots).

Primary care capitation

Payment is fixed (normally per month) per member, and is made regardless of utilization. The services covered by capitation may vary. Under full capitation the physician is at risk for all medical services, including referral services and hospitalization. However, it is important to realize that this remains (at present) a relatively uncommon payment method in the USA, a much more common approach being for only certain service elements to be capitated.

Typically, under primary care capitation, the PCP is capitated for a fixed list of services. Withholds for referral and hospital costs exceeding a set amount per member per month are also common to discourage inappropriate referrals and/or shifting of workload. Other services are reimbursed on a fee-for-service basis. This payment method is relatively popular and this mixture of capitation and fee-for-service goes some way to addressing those critics of full or global capitation who claim that quality will suffer as providers limit patient access to make money. This remains the principal concern of critics of capitation systems in general (outside of physician groups who – correctly – suspect that capitation will ultimately be used to attempt a reduction in doctors' incomes).

Capitation systems as a whole are designed to eliminate traditional fee-for-service incentives and can also transfer much of the financial risk of claims fluctuation to the capitated provider (in this case the doctor). Although the argument that quality is at risk has substance it should also be borne in mind that in the USA the public has a choice of plan. Substandard care is likely to be punished both in the marketplace and the courts. However, there remains a concern that for certain members this will be too late and that their loss will go beyond that of mere disappointment with the services on offer! It is against this background that full or global capitation is examined.

Full/global capitation

This technique creates the most dramatic financial incentives to control the cost of medical services. The physician would receive a capitation rate covering all services. Typically, the actual payments for hospital and referral services would be made by the HMO and deducted from the capitation. The PCPs will receive whatever funds are left over from the capitation pool after all claims are paid. As previously noted, passing risk to physicians also reduces the financial risk to the funding body (in this case an HMO). The idea of using payment systems to distribute risk has not had much exposure in the UK literature, and is worth serious examination. In this context it is worth remembering that capitation is by no means a one-sided system, designed solely to disadvantage the physician. In the USA passing financial risk to providers also means reducing the possible gains to the HMO if experience is more favourable than expected. For instance, if claims were significantly below budget (forgetting for the moment cause and effect), an HMO would experience the greatest gains if providers were not capitated.

The same logic could apply within the NHS should GP and/or practice reimbursement be capitated in a similar manner to that described above.

Capitation payments are often adjusted for the demographic profile of members and some may go further to reflect the current acuity, or case mix of the membership. As a result of this, and the use of other adjustments (risk pools, withholds etc. which are explained later in this chapter), the formula by which physicians are actually reimbursed can attain a considerable degree of complexity. The movement to capitation payment and the obstacles it has to overcome are considered more fully later in this chapter. An interesting perspective on the increasing trend towards capitation is that at one level it represents a partial confession by insurers and regulators that they have performed poorly in managing costs. All the traditional methods of cost control – education, audit, utilization review, pre-authorization, discount purchasing etc. – have ultimately proved inadequate to manage, much less reduce the cost of health care, and raise questions about the need for such an infrastructure in a capitated environment. At its most basic, capitation is akin to saying 'here's the money, you control utilization'. The same analysis could be made for the UK with regard to the drive to move all purchasing decisions to GPs.

Hospital payment strategies

According to Kongstvedt, writing in the USA, 'it is axiomatic that medical services are bought at the margin. As with purchasing an automobile or furniture, it is unusual to pay the sticker price.'[21] In contrast, the central principle of NHS pricing as stated in financial guidance is that 'cost should equal price'.[30]

In the USA, hospitals, like physicians, have traditionally been paid on a fee-for-service basis with all its associated problems. Once again, managed care organizations attempt to create payment strategies that promote cost containment by passing risk for excessive utilization to the hospitals. The primary payment methods (involving progressively greater risk transfer) are:

- discounted charges
- per diems
- per stay
- capitation.

Discount from charges

Unlike the case of physician services, discounted charge based payments for hospitals are still quite popular in the USA. This is partly due to the fact that there is little standardization in the services billed by hospitals – making it more difficult to develop a maximum fee-per-service, partly because of the industry's familiarity with this charge method, and partly due to inertia and resistance from the hospitals to change. However, the same problems apply as were previously noted when this method of payment to physicians was discussed. It neither rewards low-cost hospitals nor penalizes high-cost ones, nor does it give the hospital much incentive to control utilization.

In Sentara's case examples can be found of discounted charges being operated in conjunction with some form of withhold in anticipation of the hospital keeping its utilization of services within a preset target. Unfortunately (but unsurprisingly) NHS trusts have proven extremely resistant to the idea of sharing risk on utilization of their services. Generally it is perceived to be in the best interests of the provider to encourage activity – as this normally generates income – particularly as many providers have excess capacity. At the same time it suits many providers to claim that they have little control over referrals and hence waiting lists and to leave the responsibility for them with purchasers. Excess capacity is an even greater problem for most US hospitals but waiting-lists are not – perhaps making them somewhat more amenable to risk-sharing proposals.

Whatever the cause, the trends in referrals to the secondary sector are going in different directions when the two countries are compared. In the USA, typically these indicators are dropping – days of care per thousand members, inpatient admissions per thousand – with the possible exception of ambulatory care. In stark contrast NHS hospital activity is up but reductions in waiting-lists often seem modest.

The position in Wales can be used to illustrate this. The total number of inpatients and day cases (in thousands) had risen from 611.2 in 1991/2 to 765.6 by 1994/5. This increase in reported activity of 154 000 cases was matched by a reduction in total waiting-lists of just 868 cases (Table 4.1). However, if we take the latest figures in Table 4.1 (June 1996) and compare them with the figures for September 1992 (the lowest reported waiting-list) we can demonstrate that the waiting-list has actually increased by 5944 cases. Clearly, perception of the scale of the problem is influenced by the years being used as a reference point, but however one looks at Table 4.1 the results are less than impressive.

Table 4.1: Welsh total waiting-lists (including fundholding)

	30.9.91	30.9.92	31.3.93	31.3.94	30.9.94	31.3.95	30.9.95	31.3.96	30.6.96
Inpatients	52 461	44 014	43 055	43 821	42 744	42 926	41 842	39 941	40 210
Day cases	10 970	12 741	14 134	17 148	16 640	19 457	20 065	20 890	22 489
Outpatients/ day cases	63 431	56 755	57 189	60 969	59 384	62 473	61 907	60 831	62 699
Outpatients	96 078	1 130 411	118 853	125 301	131 407	114 308	116 770	95 921	107 089

Source: Welsh office

Dyfed Powys Health Authority's position reflects the above. Between 1993/4 and 1995/6 total inpatients and day-case activity (including fund-holders) rose from 88 845 cases to 98 249 (an increase of 9404 cases at 10.58%), yet the total waiting-list went from 8291 to 9159 (a rise of 868 cases or 10.46%).

A partial explanation lies in the growth of emergency admissions which is an issue throughout the UK (although its impact is not uniformly felt). In Scotland, emergency admissions increased by 45% between 1981 and 1994. This represented an annual increase of about 3% rising to over 5% in 1993 and 1994 (and probably 1995). The article from which these figures are quoted referred to other studies from which it was concluded that only 2% of the increase could be explained by population aging (Capewell S (1996) The continuing rise in emergency admissions. *BMJ*. **312**: 991–2).

Wales has recorded annual fluctuations in general medical emergency admissions over the last three years, but a general rise remains the norm: in 1994 there was a 3% increase; in 1995 there was a 9% increase, and in 1996 the increase was 2%.

The factors leading to increased activity and persistent waiting-lists are likely to be so varied as to defy a simple explanation. For example, Dyfed has seen activity going up across a spectrum of specialties – some of which have short or non-existent waiting-lists, such as radiotherapy and paediatrics, and are not normally bound together as displaying the same dynamics for referral into hospital as, say, general medicine or geriatrics. Activity at the regional 'centres of excellence' has increased, sometimes dramatically. Are we to conclude that people have suddenly developed a startling range of exotic diseases and suffered from a small explosion in the incidence of cancer? If so, why is this not being noted in the professional journals? Surely it is naïve to believe that reimbursement mechanisms have not had some influence. This issue is looked at again later in the chapter.

Using discounts from charges as a method of payment may seem alien to those charged with NHS contracting but on reflection a typical contract between health authority and NHS trust is effectively one where specialty-based charges are agreed (Appendix III). The resistance of hospitals to the standardization of service and charges inherent in prospective payment systems (DRGs/HRGs) means that this reimbursement method effectively suffers from the same flaws as its American counterpart. Where NHS payers (health authorities and fundholders) are able to negotiate price variations compared to other payers these can be seen effectively as a discount on charges. The relative lack of interest shown by NHS policy-makers on the impact of various reimbursement methodologies on provider behaviour is somewhat puzzling. It does mean that there remains considerable scope for refinement and reform and in this context the various reimbursement methodologies outlined here represent the principal options.

Per diem reimbursement

This is a common form of reimbursement by which the hospital is paid a fixed amount a day regardless of its actual level of expenditure on services.

One survey found that some 15–20% of hospital revenues were paid by per diem compared with only 7% via capitation.[31] The rest came about from DRGs and regular/discounted charges. The two biggest problems with the per diem method of reimbursement are:

- as part of the 'fee-for-service family' it does little to discourage admissions to the hospital

- it creates an incentive to increase length of stay, since the facility is paid more the longer a patient remains.

The means by which HMOs try to counter this and other payment systems' adverse incentives are examined in the next chapter but it should be noted that there is a body within the managed care industry which very much favours a per diem payment system. Their reasoning is that they will typically have in place an infrastructure of utilization review and on-site case coordinators. The latter, in particular, are focused on ensuring lengths of stay are appropriate and quickly identifying bottlenecks. Inappropriate stays can be denied payment, whilst physicians working within the managed care programme (remember that both PCPs and specialists are reimbursed separately from the hospital) can be given incentives to reduce lengths of stay. Under a per diem system, savings resulting from the reductions in the length of stay would go to the HMO (and in all probability also partly to participating physicians). In any form of prospective payment system the major beneficiary would be the hospital.

Variations on this basic approach include the negotiation of multiple sets of per diem charges based on service type (e.g. obstetrics, intensive care, neonatal intensive care and rehabilitation) and a sliding scale which reduces per diem rates as volume grows (reflecting the economics at work of marginal cost/marginal revenue). Finally, a differential by day in hospital (reflecting the fact that most hospitalizations are more expensive on the first day) might be agreed. It is worth remembering that negotiating such a payment process is one thing. The organization's ability to administer it may be another thing altogether.

Should this approach to reimbursement be applied to the NHS? Caution is advised for at least three reasons:

- adequate monitoring of per diem payment systems implies the existence of a medical care management and information infrastructure which simply is not in place in the NHS

- NHS consultants are hospital employees and therefore have different incentives than their free agent counterparts in the USA

- if you can accurately predict the number and mix of cases you could calculate a proposed per diem rate. It is therefore very important that one has a predictable volume and case mix. Both these areas are very volatile in the NHS at present – even for fundholders.

Finally, there is simply more than one way to skin this particular cat. Providing you are prepared to take a medium-term view, prospective payment systems (DRGs, HRGs and chargeable procedures) can be used to reflect changes in length of stay and cost. These factors can be taken into account in reviewing next year's reimbursement rate. Allowing hospitals to make gains on a year-by-year basis through innovation and adjusting accordingly seems desirable. The biggest problem is likely to be caused where hospitals are not allowed to keep any of these gains. In this case they may decide that further innovation will only serve ultimately to reduce reimbursement levels further. As always the existence or absence of viable competitors will be important in determining provider responses to any particular reimbursement system.

Per stay reimbursement

With these contracts, hospitals are paid a fixed amount per stay regardless of actual resource use or length of stay. The UK has some familiarity with this contracting method as Wales is introducing DRGs whilst chargeable procedures and HRGs are variations on the same reimbursement philosophy. HRGs constitute the reimbursement methodology of choice in England, although the timetable for their implementation as the means of mediating contractual relationships is less than clear. In the USA, the principal per stay payment methodology used by managed care companies remains the DRG.

As previously noted, per stay contracting is not favoured by some US organizations on the grounds that the cost savings associated with length of stay reductions accrue to the provider and not the purchaser. However, this argument holds less weight if one has confidence about the level at which DRG rates have been set. The other principal concern is with 'DRG creep' (a propensity on the part of the provider to code clinical activity in such a way as to maximize reimbursement). This can be countered by undertaking coding audits and then imposing significant penalties to discourage abuse. This is the preferred method of federal and state agencies but may not be particularly attractive to the NHS for three reasons:

- its coding base is generally poor. Providers are still able to increase their case-mix base legitimately through more accurate coding

- purchasers have relatively little experience in 'policing' coding through audit and the environment is not conducive to diverting resources into such 'non-clinical' activities

- there is already considerable resistance to the imposition of financial penalties within contracts by providers and no counterbalancing enthusiasm for such disciplinary measures from policy makers. In this context it has already been noted that the Labour Party in particular is promoting collaborative approaches between purchasers and providers on contract issues.

DRGs remain a widely used reimbursement system in the USA. Sentara, like many managed care companies, utilize them and they remain the payment methodology of the federal and state programmes – Medicare and Medicaid. As in the UK, prospective payment systems have their advocates and detractors. The debate in the USA lies less in principles – such as the clinical assumptions underlying their construction – as in the pragmatic issue of whether this payment tool offers payers the best way to save money whilst ensuring quality is maintained. The UK, in contrast, has spent a great deal of time arguing the relative merits of DRGs vs HRGs vs chargeable procedures in terms of their clinical validity and usefulness for audit – reflecting an underlying concern as to their acceptability to doctors – at the expense of much consideration as to their impact on the contracting process.

Many NHS hospital executives and almost as many purchasers are 'against' the use of DRGs as a reimbursement tool, but this does not mean they necessarily support other case-mix methodologies. For many, the real objection is to change – particularly when the change in question may disadvantage their organization financially. This is understandable, to a degree. However, against this mindset no methodology can be wholly satisfactory. Managers in the USA, whilst no less mindful of their organization's financial position, tend to see change as both inevitable and the harbinger of opportunity.

Nevertheless, there remains spasmodic enthusiasm for case-mix-based contracting from UK policy makers and periodic edicts to the service to move forward on this basis.[32] Whilst this may be commendable, the lack of resources, and understanding to take forward such an initiative is not. To date, all these initiatives have foundered on three major obstacles:

- lack of an in-depth understanding of the role of case mix in operating a market

- lack of resources

- unwillingness to face up to the issues case mix will highlight.

The lack of an in-depth understanding of the role of case mix in operating a market is especially apparent amongst the NHS's most senior personnel. Their modus operandi remains rooted in managing health care as a political enterprise (see also Chapter 7).

Once the initial flush of monies associated with the resource management initiative[33] was exhausted, few additional resources were made available and then only on a haphazard basis (see also Chapter 6). This on/off approach has been (and remains) an almost complete waste of time and money. Moving to case-mix contracting is not going to happen in a timely or coordinated fashion with staff trying to undertake such a complex process on a part-time basis, or viewing it as yet another 'project'. The initiative needs the most senior public commitment, adequate pump-priming, and a phased timetable for its implementation. If additional staff are not to be made available, then it should be made clear that an organization's staffing should observe 'Sutton's law' and 'go where the money is' – an organizational principle that should not require the introduction of case-mix contracting to be acted upon but is too rarely put into practice in the NHS.

As previously indicated, unwillingness to face up to the issues that the case mix will highlight is the greatest obstacle to change. There is a saying that 'if you do not wish to be a victim of change – anticipate it'. There are occasions that one might think the operating maxim of the NHS is 'if you do not wish to be a victim of change – pretend the issues that arise do not exist'. As noted in the first chapter, having initiated the most radical reform of the British system of health care in over 40 years, much time and energy has been spent by successive Conservative governments avoiding its consequences and denying its impact. It is in this environment that resistance to case-mix contracting can best be understood.

Sentara's use of DRGs

Within Sentara the debate centres around whether DRGs allow hospitals too much freedom to make profit – the per diem debate previously referred to. Sentara's use of DRGs largely mimics Medicare's – that is, they use it as a standard reimbursement methodology. All of the company's hospitals get paid the same amount for the DRG in question, regardless of their particular costs. This was a corporate decision. It is worth remembering that not all of Sentara's hospitals will have the same costs. The tertiary facility is always likely to have a higher set of both fixed and variable costs and the four acute hospitals have significantly different occupancy rates. In this respect the company's reimbursement policy is tougher than both Medicare's and Medicaid's as they adjust payments on a number of factors, depending on location (rural or inner city), kind of hospital (teaching or otherwise), local price index etc. Sentara's view is that some of these factors are already in the case-mix weight (i.e. heart transplants are only undertaken in tertiary centres), and that at the system level one Sentara facility's loss is another's gain: a view reinforced by three of the company's four hospitals operating as one division.

One significant anomaly, however, is that Optima and Sentara Health Plan operate different payment rates by having slightly different case weights for the same DRG. There is no logical explanation for this in terms of DRG methodology. Rather it is a historical anomaly, brought about largely by attempts to pacify the hospitals and physicians who 'felt' that SHP patients had a tendency to be sicker. This would also act as an inducement for providers to participate in the managed care programme. At the time of writing this looked set to disappear into a standard (lower) rate, but it is a good example of the pragmatic attitude of commercial management.

In discussions with both US executives and academics, the reluctance of UK policy makers to adopt a consistent contracting methodology and uniform reimbursement rates is viewed with some puzzlement. A typical question is: 'How are you hoping to operate a market successfully when you have no clarity on your currency?' Most American purchasers would love to have the potential for leverage and muscle power that the NHS Management Executive has, and they are typically baffled by the lack of will to use it. As one executive observed: 'You could screw down the Providers so tight, year on year, using a common case-mix methodology that they would be screaming blue murder'.

As previously noted this is probably one of the principal reasons – alongside an inadequate understanding of market mechanisms and the methodologies themselves – that it is not happening. A compromise solution might be to adopt elements of the Canadian funding system[34] for hospitals, where global budgets for each hospital are based on a mixture of historical and projected case mix. Whilst it is difficult to see such a system operating in the increasingly fragmented purchasing environment of fundholding this may be the payment system of choice of a Labour government.

Sentara are beginning to negotiate contracts known as 'bundled' case rates or 'package pricing' in areas such as obstetrics and cardiac surgery. These combine institutional and professional charges into a single pay-ment as well as preoperative and postoperative care. The former already effectively occurs in the UK where the hospital charge includes all hospital medical staff costs. Package pricing – which could include all elements of care including community services – is of more interest. Currently, the typical community component of a provider contract is a cost and activity 'black hole'. There would appear to be considerable potential for the development of package pricing within both health care systems, although it would seem wise in the NHS for all parties to obtain greater familiarity with more orthodox reimbursement methodologies and costing systems before attempting such an innovative contracting approach.

The same might also be said for 'blended' case rates, which can be used both to control costs and to influence delivery patterns by making explicit the type of procedure mix one expects to see. This is particularly attractive where clinicians appear to have some leeway as to the rate and type of procedure performed (as illustrated by MPV analysis). In the USA, the most common use of blended case rates is in obstetrics. The expected reimbursement for each type of delivery is multiplied by the expected (or desired) percentage of utilization. For example, a case rate for vaginal delivery might be $1900 and for caesarean section $2400. Utilization is set at 90% vaginal and 10% caesarean section. In this example the blended case rate is $1900 \times 0.8 = $1520; $2400 \times 0.2 = $480; $1520 + $480 = $2000.

The typical NHS contract for obstetrics sets a *de facto* blended rate, with none of the preliminary work-up. The specialty cost per case will include all births regardless of their delivery method, costs and outcome. Undertaking a thorough analysis of current practice, and then agreeing a blended rate based on the practice pattern one wishes to see, allows the contracting methodology to become a force for change. However, such a reimbursement mechanism depends on adequate staffing resources to devise and monitor the contract, and on accurate information being readily available.

Finally, some managed care companies also operate bundled charges for ambulatory procedures – what the NHS typically classifies as day cases. All the various charges are bundled into one single charge for all procedures, using historical data. Extreme caution is advised for anyone contemplating using this technique in the UK. The existence of waiting-lists and the varying ability of consultants to 'cherry pick' low case-mix cases off it, coupled with opportunities to reclassify outpatient activity to day cases, makes this reimbursement method open to manipulation. The capacity for abuse is significantly reduced for fundholders (who typically have a good idea as to the structure – and exercise greater control – of their waiting-lists), but even here the current dynamism of waiting-lists and clinical coding make this a relatively high-risk contracting strategy. Conversely, if purchasers exercised direct control of waiting-lists including the order in which patients were treated (which entails significant erosion of the traditional clinical autonomy of hospital consultants), the risk would shift to the hospital as the bundled charge might no longer adequately reflect the actual case mix.

Capitation payments

As previously noted, of all the payment systems for hospitals so far described, capitation payments is the only one – of itself – that creates a significant incentive for the hospital both to reduce the admissions, length of stay and resource use. In the USA, capitating hospitals entails making a per member per month (PMPM) payment for a defined population with some further adjustments likely for demographic profile, acuity, risk-pooling etc. The money is usually paid monthly, and while it may vary based on such factors as age and sex of the patients, it is independent of the actual volume or cost of the services rendered. If a hospital cannot provide the service itself (and therefore makes a tertiary referral), the cost for such care is deducted from the capitation payment.

Ancillary services payment systems

As much as one third of health care costs in the USA are not categorized under either hospital inpatient or physician services. These include out-patient care (which in the USA includes much day-case surgery), drugs and appliances. In the case of the former, the use of discounted charges was once popular, partly to encourage such services as a substitute to in-patient care, and partly because there was no commonly used methodology for categorizing claims. These are now increasingly being replaced by procedure-based reimbursement methodologies based on the intensity of the services performed.

In the case of prescription drugs, the use of discount arrangements and a set formulary is common. Cost containment in the drug arena is a growing issue (particularly for the growing elderly population) and both HMOs and insurance companies tend to exclude drug benefits from their plans on the grounds that to do otherwise makes the product either uneconomic to operate or unattractive to potential members (due to cost) or both! As in other areas capitation is being introduced. HMOs may also try to agree preferred provider status to a particular retail pharmacy chain (examples might be Boots plc in the UK, or Revco in the USA) and try to steer its members to these companies. In return, it gets a discount on drug charges.

Contracting for mental health, learning disabilities and substance abuse services

The development of adequate contractual relationships in the field of mental health, learning disabilities and substance abuse, so as to ensure value for money and quality services, has proved problematical on both sides of the Atlantic. At its root lies a common set of problems, centred around high rates of unexplained medical practice variation, a dearth of commissioned research on both treatment process and outcomes, and a lack of an adequate case-mix methodology. Of the latter, the barriers to developing a case-mix methodology as a predictive tool for resource use are formidable. Many problems in the areas of mental health, learning disabilities and substance abuse tend to be chronic and recurrent, requiring periodic and sometimes intensive treatment. Diagnostic categories do not lend themselves to systematic utilization management with expected lengths of stay and treatment protocols for each diagnosis. Both causes and progression of the 'diseases' in question elude a ready explanation (knowledge on the workings of the human mind remains largely guesswork), and the result is often a disturbingly large range of treatment approaches. A cynic might say that the cost consequence and course of treatment for a particular type of mental illness are more likely to be predictable, not by reference to any diagnosis, but by observing whether the clinicians treating the case had a preference for talking, shocking or drugging their respective charges! To this methodological wilderness can be added the unfortunate observation that these areas of illness get less attention than perhaps they deserve because of their relative stigmatization and resultant marginalization by society.

Substantive efforts at managing mental health and substance abuse treatments – and costs in particular – are more visible in the HMO industry than in the UK. Even that effort is incomplete as the area of interest usually is limited to outpatient activities (on the basis that inpatient treatment is often not covered in the plan's benefits), but a review of HMO activities in this area is nevertheless useful.

Many traditional insurers have been wary of providing any coverage for these areas. Likewise, some HMOs have looked to limiting exposure to that required for compliance within the HMO act. Initially this meant there was no requirement to cover inpatient care, recurrent chronic conditions or chemical dependency, but generalizations in this area have to be tempered by the knowledge that different states require different levels of benefits.

Over time the process of underwriting and managing these services has developed into a niche industry in its own right – hence Sentara's particular organizational structure can be seen as part of a general industry trend. Covered benefits have expanded as insurers have grown more confident of their ability to manage such services and consumer demand has grown.

The insurance industry has looked to develop specialized techniques to manage costs and quality in this field (NHS purchasers may wish to reflect whether either their infrastructure or contracts reflect this need for specialist skills and techniques). Interestingly, the focus of health authorities and HMOs in relation to these services is likely to be quite different. Health authorities typically devote most time to looking at the institutional elements – concerned as they are with the closure of large hospitals, etc. – and reflecting the traditional power base of consultant psychiatrists. Contracting for non-institutional services and outpatient settings usually receives scant attention. HMOs are much more likely to be looking at the other end of the prism (a characteristic likely to be shared with many NHS fundholders). In doing so, they are helped by the fact that many hospitals dealing with mental health and learning disabilities are owned and operated by the state, and the HMO has no particular mandate to take forward a government-inspired 'policy' on mental health as is the case with UK health authority purchasers. Indeed, the concept is hardly applicable to the US system of health care. As a result, the specialized managed care programmes for this area have a greater focus on non-institutional services. According to Anderson and Berlant[35] this specialist care has its foundations in promoting four components of clinical treatment:

- alternatives to psychiatric hospitalization
- alternatives to restrictive treatment for substance abuse
- goal-directed psychotherapy
- crisis intervention.

To this might be added a realization that non-clinical support may be a cost-effective solution for some people (i.e. ensuring that members can get appropriate advice on money or childcare issues which, if left untouched, might present as a health problem – e.g. depression and drug abuse). Finally, a real concern for obtaining member feedback as part of the quality assurance process is normal.

It makes some sense to look at the above in terms of benefit plan design as this is the starting point for any managed care programme, and in particular the question of coverage limits and incentives. In doing so, the principal difference between the traditional role of the NHS as purchaser and that of an HMO once again becomes apparent – that is the HMO's desire and ability to limit exposure through its benefit plans, a facility not available to health authorities, but with some relevance to fundholders. This feature of US health care makes the provision of seamless continuity of care extremely difficult to achieve (presupposing all parties wish such a state of affairs). It remains to be seen if the NHS reforms will result in a further fragmentation of responsibilities in an area where patients are particularly vulnerable – there already being a fundamental discontinuity caused by the division of duties between local government and health authorities. As such, any positive lessons (as opposed to warnings) coming from the managed care movement will tend to lie in the mechanisms of contract review and quality control. This would help to bring greater accountability on providers for their actions and start the process of determining value for money in a field whose practitioners have historically had great difficulty in accepting any form of quantitative measurement of their services.

Coverage limits

Coverage limits act as plan safeguards (that is they are designed to protect the company, not the patient, from excessive costs). The concept is no different for mental health than for other areas of health care and can include a cap on days of inpatient care, outpatient visits, levels of care, types of treatment and even specific diagnoses. Likewise, deductibles and copayments (particularly for out-of-plan providers) are likely to be a plan feature, perhaps with a maximum dollar limit on lifetime costs for an individual ($125 000, for example).

Given the chronic and unpredictable nature of much mental illness and substance abuse, it might well be concluded that the insurance market represents a particularly poor mechanism for ensuring adequate services to those in need – a view which the author shares. A comprehensive managed care programme should include access to different levels of care (individual, group treatment, non-residential care, crisis intervention, community services, inpatient etc.) and a range of providers (counsellors, psychologists, psychiatric nurses, psychiatrists and psychotherapists). Despite this, an insurance-based system has intrinsic limitations as a means of ensuring comprehensive coverage for all individuals. In their favour, good HMOs are able to point to a network of providers based on some form of needs assessment for their members rather than expecting people to fit into a predetermined set of services dictated by vested medical interests. The latter is a description of services familiar to many in the UK, although, in fairness, if the NHS rarely reaches the 'highs' of best practice US style, nor does it plumb its 'lows'.

Utilization management

Any form of utilization or case management demonstrated by the US system is likely to be valuable to NHS purchasers as it is almost non-existent at present as it relates to the NHS purchasing function. In the USA the conventional wisdom is that: 'utilisation review conducted by non-specialised staff with general medical background(s) was ineffective when applied to mental health/substance abuse cases.'[21] This explains the growth of 'niche' companies employing specialized staff applying specific utilization criteria. These techniques include:

- preadmission certification of inpatient cases
- concurrent review of inpatient and residential cases
- concurrent review of designated outpatient cases
- case management
- use of a selected, specialized network of providers.

The latter point is considered particularly important by commentators such as Anderson and Berlant.[35] This view is likely to find favour with NHS managers who would prescribe to the widely held (if rarely stated) view that there are proportionately more poor clinicians in this area of medicine. Health authorities or fundholders thinking of setting up specialized utilization review (UR) programmes need to consider that the most effective HMOs would typically employ credentialled reviewers with experience in the principal treatment settings and who in turn have access to high-level clinical input to provide appropriate back-up. In NHS purchasing, too few public health medicine/nursing staff can claim the appropriate experience.

Case management

In the USA, comprehensive managed care in the areas of mental health, substance abuse and learning disabilities now emphasizes the role of case management as the most effective means of ensuring quality, cost-effective care (along with the selection of appropriate providers). Case management should look beyond a discrete episode of care and encompass patient advocacy. Although a familiar concept to psychiatry, it takes on a new dimension when applied to the purchasing of such services. When the principal elements of case management are examined, it becomes apparent that it implies a degree of 'management' of the patient and service delivery which most NHS agencies (on both sides of the purchaser–provider divide) would find unsettling, including:

- the promotion of an accurate diagnosis and effective treatment for members

- ensuring efficient use of resources

- preventing relapse (and encouraging compliance with treatment regimens)

- monitoring care and taking action on substandard services.

NHS purchasers are unlikely to have the resources to undertake such case management on anything other than a highly selected basis. However, the case for such proactive management is indicated by the continued concern about the adequacy of community care* and the proper targeting of the resources available to those in greatest need. These issues are clearly interconnected; on the first issue, the Mental Health (Patients in the Community) Act, 1995, was enacted largely as an attempt to ensure that patients discharged to the community continue to comply with their drug/treatment regimens and that the 'duty of care' relationship between mental health professionals and their clients extends beyond the hospital grounds. With regard to the second issue, an analysis of the caseload of community psychiatric nurses (CPNs) is particularly illuminating. Recent studies have confirmed the suspicion that, left to their own devices, community mental health teams have a tendency to gravitate towards patients with less severe and/or more treatable conditions. Whilst it is understandable that many staff prefer to work with those patients most likely to return to full health and demonstrating fewer antisocial characteristics, it is yet another example of the inverse care law. Fundholding may accentuate this disparity as GPs use their control of community psychiatric resources to reduce their own workloads. Peck[37] noted this perception that:

> Many GP fundholders are not targeting their resources on the long term and seriously mentally ill as prescribed by government policy and that in extending the amount of care purchased for people outside of those two priority groups, GP fundholders may be drawing scarce professional resources, particularly Community Psychiatric Nurses, away from those two groups

*The *Economist*[36] reported in August 1996 that over the past year and a half there have been 14 reports of inquiries into murders by mentally ill people and there are another two dozen in preparation.

and into working with people who have less severe, if still significant, mental health problems.

This view is supported by an Audit Commission report which stated:[38]

> Some [community mental health] teams were found to give priority to people with severe problems but others work mainly with those who have lesser problems. This lack of focus on those with severe problems is worrying. In districts where teams spend almost all of their time with people with lesser problems, many of those with severe mental illness and long term problems may not be receiving a service.

The report went on to make a striking indictment of current practice by observing that:

> In many districts the CPNs had a smaller proportion of people with severe mental illness on their caseloads than any other professional group, despite the professions having been created largely to help people with long term mental illness. In one district the CPNs saw a lower proportion of people in Category A (the most severely mentally ill) than did the social workers. Nationally, the CPNs have shifted their working patterns away from those with severe problems and a quarter of CPNs do not have a single person with schizophrenia on their caseload.

In summary, whilst there may be a wide range of people who would benefit from specialist mental health service input, the principal focus must remain the severely mentally ill. This is as much a purchaser responsibility as any mental health professional's, and the current monitoring arrangements are inadequate. It is no longer sufficient (if it ever was) for NHS purchasers simply to hand over monies effectively as a block contract and say 'we trust you to deliver the right services', rationalizing that to do otherwise takes too much time and effort.

Given the limited resources available to NHS purchasers (in terms of both money and manpower), it is unrealistic to try and establish an HMO-type monitoring infrastructure. Instead, it is proposed that the NHS ensures that contracts contain quality specifications which detail key deliverables for the service, which are subsequently monitored, so that action can be taken on any shortfalls. These will necessarily have to be few in number, but the important thing will be to communicate that the purchaser is not some passive middleman for transferring monies from the treasury to the service, but has a view about the services that should be delivered and ensures that the provider(s) do so. For example, the purchaser should set out the expected case mix dealt with by community mental health teams and during the year undertake (with the provider) audit on a random sample basis. On the issue of clinical audit itself, the purchaser should be particularly proactive – setting a number of topics and insisting it sees results.

Purchasers should be making greater efforts to establish user views about the service. Where it becomes clear that there are substandard clinicians, the provider should be given a limited time to tackle the problem. Where no progress is made, purchasers should refuse to buy services from named individuals (in the same way that it should increasingly decide who can and cannot undertake certain surgical procedures and medical treatments in acute trusts). There are far too many substandard clinicians in this field of medicine and purchasers need to recognize that it is their responsibility (as much, if not more, than a trust's) to identify those individuals and do something about it.

Because too few purchasers have ready access to high-quality mental health professionals within their own organization (a problem which is increasing with each year of management cuts) they must work to pool resources between them. The NHS neither wants nor can afford a bureaucratic care management system at purchaser level, but it should develop an adequate infrastructure to undertake periodic case management reviews to highlight deficiencies in service provision. If health authorities, in particular, were more effective in this area, it is likely that some of the scandals that we have all read about (and, unfortunately, will continue to see) would be averted.

Adjusting payments for risk-sharing

There are a number of refinements and adjustments made to a typical payment scheme which do not really fall into either the capitation or fee-for-service philosophies. Most of these adjustments are there to limit specific risks (i.e. risks which are deemed to be uncontrollable or not appropriate to transfer).

The need to account for, and seek protection from, the costs associated with 'catastrophic cases', results in special financing arrangements. Unforeseen and rare occurrence high-cost cases are part and parcel of modern medicine. Protection from catastrophic claims has a number of benefits as it reduces claims fluctuations and stabilizes cash flow, whilst avoiding the unpleasant experience of a single case wiping out the various parties' funds and/or profits.

The following are common examples of payment adjustments made to protect against catastrophic risk:

- physician capitations are commonly supplemented by fee-for-service type payments for patients whose costs exceed an annual preset limit. For example, an HMO might pay a percentage (say 90%) of all primary care charges exceeding $4000 in a year for any patient covered under a primary care capitation scheme. Note that the HMO only pays a percentage and not the whole amount, thus aiming to retain the physicians' interest in controlling utilization for the cases in question

- when amounts withheld from physicians are paid back based on service usage, the costs of a particular individual patient's care may be excluded from the performance goals set, if those costs exceed a predetermined amount. For example, a limit of charges against the pool per case might be set at $20 000 to reduce the chance that such cases will wipe out the pool monies and hence the physicians' withhold

- hospital contracts often have an 'outlier' provision for cases requiring exceptional lengths of stay and/or costs. Once again these are likely to be paid at a percentage of normal rates.

Risk pools

Payment adjustments can take a number of forms and impact on, and help create, risk-pooling agreements. These are agreements between two or more parties (HMOs, PCPs, specialists and hospitals) to share risk on certain performance targets being met. Each party may be 'at risk' for a different percentage (often meant to represent their respective ability to control the expenditures in question) and they will receive payouts from the pool or lose the pooled funds based on their respective percentages.

Risk pools and the use of reinsurance (see below) serve two purposes. They aim to set risk at a controllable level, but they should also keep the relevant parties interested in the cost consequences of such cases. This is an underdeveloped area in the NHS where the statutorily determined divisions between GPs, trusts, health authorities and other agencies such as social services have encouraged each party to consider its finances (and financial relationships) in isolation to each other. In a closed-loop funding system such as the NHS operates within, this borders on self-delusion. At some point the political expediency of ignoring such issues is likely to be less than the benefits of addressing real risk-sharing. Here American experience and techniques are likely to be useful. One example is the use of 'risk corridors' as set out below. (The term 'provider' can mean PCP – the HMO's GPs – and hospital specialists, as well as the hospital itself.)

- a target cost is set per member per month. The provider is responsible for the costs, or gains up to ± 10% of the target

- above 110% and below 90% the excess is split on a pro rata basis (i.e. 50/50)

- there would normally be an overall limit on losses (i.e. stop-loss).

Another form of risk-pooling is to set a quota share on the level of control each party has on the type of service being provided. The steps are as follows:

- determine level of control by type of service

- assign a quota share percentage for each party reflecting control level

- compare actual results to target sets by type of service

- providers responsible for their share of gain/loss of each type of service pool.

An example of a quota share from the USA (where physicians are generally not hospital employees and are billed separately) is as follows:

- assume two pools

  - hospital
  - physician

- hospitals retain 90% control of hospital pool, 10% to physicians

- physicians retain 90% control of physician pool, 10% to hospitals

- target hospital pool   – $75.00 per member per month

- target physician pool – $75.00 per member per month

- actual hospital pool   – $65.00 per member per month

- actual physician pool – $85.00 per member per month.

Settlements

In any settlement, the following conditions apply:

- hospital retains 90% of $10.00 gain in hospital pool

- physician retains 10% of $10.00 gain in hospital pool

- hospital retains 10% of $10.00 loss in physician pool

- physician retains 90% of $10.00 loss in physician pool.

As previously noted, NHS hospital management and medical staff prefer to distance themselves from issues relating to patient utilization – claiming minimal control over referral rates, treatments and costs. The documented national variations in all three areas belie this convenient abdication of responsibility. Quota shares may help to reflect the various levels of influence each party can bring to bear. The idea could be extended as a means of sharing risk between primary and secondary care, particularly if total GP purchasing/commissioning becomes the norm.

The explosion of NHS hospital activity in the 1990s has already been noted. Consider further this example of radiotherapy treatment at a hospital in South Wales for patients from Dyfed (which has a stable population base). Inpatient activity increased from 817 discharges and deaths to 1016 (24.3%) in just two years (1994/5–1995/6). New outpatients activity went up from a contracted activity base of 420 to an out-turn of 707 (68%) during the same period, whilst day cases rose from 230 to 386 (67%). Moreover there was no counterbalancing reduction in radiotherapy activity at other hospitals. In fact overall these went from just 47 inpatients to 58, 56 day cases to 152, and 921 new outpatient cases to 1008.

Is radiotherapy an elective treatment? The initial reaction is to dismiss such a suggestion as absurd. However, on reflection there may be a large clinical 'grey area' where the efficacy of the decision to start and stop treatment is by no means clear-cut (after all, to the layman, the decision about whether to undertake a coronary artery bypass graft or offer renal dialysis might seem a black-and-white issue, yet we find significant regional variations in the UK, and have already noted that the USA performs ten times the rate of coronary artery surgery). Is it coincidental that during the time period under observation the Calman Report[39] was issued, which emphasizes the importance of high volumes in ensuring clinical quality and good outcomes, and aims to bestow coveted 'cancer centre' status on those few hospitals that can generate such a critical clinical mass? Or was there perhaps an unexplained rise in cancer incidence, better recording of clinical activity, or a change in clinical practice? At the time of writing no one knows for sure – and interestingly, unless the initiative is taken locally, no one at the policy-making level would be likely to question this phenomenon – but it is clear where the financial risk lies. It is largely one-sided, as were the incentives. As an illustration, the base contract cost to the health authority for this one area (with the hospital in question) rose by £429 185 (25.5%) for 1996/7 in contrast to 1995/6.

Stop-loss reinsurance

There are two types of stop-loss reinsurance: specific and aggregate.

Specific stop-loss insurance limits liability to a predetermined amount for any single case during a defined time period. Aggregate stop-loss limits liability to a predetermined amount for the entire insured group for a given time period. For example, losses might be capped at 125% of expected claims. The cap may not be total. For example it is common that the stop-loss reinsurance covers most, but not all, the additional expenses (say 90%). This provides added incentive to avoid or contain such cases.

In the UK this whole area is given inadequate attention – that is the need to maintain financial reserves sufficient to cover potential adverse experiences in the utilization and cost of health care services. This area is being further complicated by the introduction of fundholding and more sophisticated contracting methodologies (insofar as case-mix-based payments implicitly acknowledge that complex cases cost more, and the traditional block contract approach whereby one gave over a sum of money – which typically had no methodological basis other than it was close to last year's payment – and told the provider to 'get on with it' is no longer a tenable means of negotiating contracts with providers).

Fundholders and more particularly the total fundholding pilots effectively act as small insurance companies, and further consideration needs to be given to the fact that fluctuations in the experience of small groups of patients cannot be predicted with any degree of accuracy. This leads one to the conclusion that the 'risk' of such uncontrollable, catastrophic claims can best be absorbed by a larger entity.

Here the US experience is relevant in two ways. First, an HMO takes care to set aside funds for such adverse cases before allocating its capitation funding. In the UK, health authorities are required to allocate funds to fundholders without any reference to the subsequent financial commitments they retain due to the scheme's regulatory framework (for example the requirement to take over the funding of cases once costs exceed £6000 total elective care costs).

Second, HMOs with member populations not dissimilar from an NHS authority see it as prudent to 'lay off' risk for particularly high-cost cases (as already explained above). This policy might be usefully adopted by those authorities which currently have a propensity for underestimating the financial impact of such cases. Inadequate financial provision has a number of negative consequences including:

- crisis actions (including cancelling planned expenditure, refusing to pay, asking providers to take immediate action to reduce costs which often result in only marginal savings but considerable pain to all parties etc.)

- continued overspending

- negotiating the costs in question downwards as a series of 'special deals' with the result that the true costs of health care for various conditions are distorted and cross-subsidization occurs.

A similar policy to that seen in the USA (with perhaps the regions acting as reinsurance agents or commercial insurers being used) would reduce the variability of the claims experience and mollify its destabilizing effects. This will be even more important if GPs eventually undertake all purchasing – given their list sizes. The current use of extra-contractual referral (ECR) budgets as a pseudo-risk management device – as well as being the catch-all budget for cases that fall outside of the normal contracts – is flawed, not least because the current regulations do not allow referrals to be refused on financial grounds. Unsurprisingly, most ECR budgets are overspending. If you wish to hold purchasers responsible for budgetary control they have to be given the means to keep expenditure within the limits set. The further liberalization of the ECR system recently announced has further undermined purchasers' ability to control costs in this area.[40] Whilst total fundholding would make this easier – after all they are making the initial referrals, if not the consultant to consultant ones (the latter typically consume the greatest resources) – it will not eliminate the problem. To the inherent problems of unpredictability and small list size need to be added the traditional expectation that someone else will provide financial assistance for exceptional cases and unforeseen expenditure. Whilst this is a role the new authorities/regions might assume, they can only do so effectively if some control mechanisms remain in force and resources are devoted to it. At present, there is no recognition by politicians that there is a problem, once again showing the dichotomy between the objectives being set for purchasers and the means available to the purchasers to achieve them.

UK applications

At first sight, US moves towards capitation seem very similar to the fundholding initiative and may even elicit the response: 'What's all the fuss about?' UK readers will probably regard the NHS as already ahead of most HMOs in terms of setting global budgets and getting GPs and hospitals to operate within them. Whilst it may be true that there is a fair amount of reticence in the US about adopting full capitation (partly because of the anticipated resistance of the powerful specialist and hospital interest groups), the American system has more radical aspects with regard to:

- the linkage between performance to plan and personal income, and from that, the direct financial risk to physicians' personal income that capitation presents

- the capitation base is standardized on a PMPM basis using a common formula. An individual practitioner's or group's historical use of resources is not part of the equation, although the sum total of PCP's past resource use has some bearing – in that HMOs attempt to base their capitation formulae on a mix of actuarial analysis and projected utilization

- most of the players operating in the US health market are commercial enterprises, financially at risk for all of the decisions they make and the contracts they sign. In contrast, it is easy to be relatively cavalier about costing and contracting issues if you believe there is an appeal process which will allow you to subvert market disciplines.

The dynamics of fundholding and the case for capitation

The importance of sound reimbursement mechanisms and in particular, of a viable system of capitation becomes more obvious when one considers the future of general practice purchasing in general, and fundholding in particular within the UK. The greater involvement of doctors in general, and GPs in particular, in the direct management of NHS resources is here to stay.

Whether fundholding as it is currently established and regulated will endure is by no means as certain. Its extension – in number of GPs and scope – may well be a temporary phenomenon. One scenario is that over time a sobering reality will lend balance to the enthusiasm of current pioneers and that a combination of well-publicized failures, financial scandals and regulatory problems will lead to the pendulum swinging back in favour of a more centralized (and more easily controlled) purchasing function. This does not preclude some form of GP commissioning (as perhaps the Labour party has in mind), but the emphasis of this model is that GP autonomy would be more limited than fundholders currently enjoy. On the general issue of GP purchasing, the particular colour of government may serve to accelerate or retard this process but there are sufficient tensions and contradictions within the current reform process to ensure that the dialectic of change continues.

Consider for a moment the state of general practice. To call it a reluctant bride in a hastily arranged marriage to the Conservative government's reforms is not only murdering a set of similes, but also seriously understates the unpreparedness, uncertainty and occasionally outright hostility to the suitor. Would anyone be surprised if an acrimonious divorce were to occur sometime in the future?

There are 32 748 GPs in the UK. As of April 1996 some 16 112 (49%) were fundholders.[41] Even the most enthusiastic advocates of the NHS reforms admit those remaining represent the GPs either most opposed, unprepared or incapable of becoming fundholders. Doctors are not a homogeneous group. With the possible exception of issues relating to their salaries and conditions of service they typically have the herding instincts of houseflies. They also display a remarkably wide range of clinical, managerial and financial competencies.

If a random sample of 100 GPs was taken, the typical distribution in terms of their interest and ability with regard to fundholding would probably be as follows.

The elite 20% will range from very good to exceptional fundholders. They will typically be interested in managerial as well as clinical issues, be innovative, and well motivated to use the scheme to benefit their patients, the NHS and the practice itself (although not necessarily in that order). They will often be pushing for change and do not feel unduly disturbed or threatened by shifts in the status quo.

Around 75% will be effectively neutral. They are likely to accept fundholding providing it does not impact too greatly on their professional lives. For many this means doing what they went into medicine for: treating patients.

The final 5% or so are the disasters waiting to happen. They in turn fall into two camps – the incompetent and the corrupt. The incompetent are in many senses the easiest to handle (providing the appropriate monitoring mechanisms are in place) because they will often also be disinterested – simply wishing others to do the work for them. However the most worrying group might be termed the 'cowboys'. Some will be incompetent, but others will show all the interest and initiative of the elite group, but with entirely selfish objectives. There are already a number of doctors – often serving the poorest and hence most vulnerable parts of the community – who appear to view their chosen vocation principally as a money-making enterprise. These are the GPs known to accident and emergency departments for their inordinate propensity to refer patients to hospital. The same doctors never seem to be available when a patient calls out of hours (instead there might be a taped message saying the doctor is busy and advising the caller to go to the accident and emergency department if they feel prompt treatment is necessary). These are the doctors who never seem to participate in audit but are well known to drug companies for their enthusiastic participation in 'sponsored' events. Everyone seems to know who they are, but no one seemingly can do anything about them.

The NHS in general and the medical profession (which fiercely defends its self-regulating status) have been ineffective in weeding out these bad apples. The above breakdown might also be applied to doctors' clinical competence – which, in the author's view, is equally poorly policed. If the utilization review techniques described later in this book were implemented in full, they might help redress the balance, but they are not sufficient in themselves to answer all the serious concerns set out in this chapter.

The above may be viewed as an attack on doctors in general and GPs in particular. This is not the author's intention. Instead the author hopes it is seen as an expression of some blunt truths – too long unspoken – whilst acknowledging that the primary care infrastructure is the greatest strength of the NHS and that the great majority of GPs are hard-working professionals who try to put the interests of their patients first.

Furthermore, GPs have made clear their discontent with their lot for some time now. This is manifesting itself through an inability to recruit trainees and the numbers opting for early retirement. Doctors in training are voting with their feet – in favour of hospital medicine. There are various reasons for this and for GP discontent in general.

Perhaps the main reason is the requirement for 24-hour cover of patients on their list, and more particularly the need to be available out of hours 'on call'. The traditional image of the single-handed family practitioner, always available for his or her patients, holds little appeal to most young doctors (the majority of whom are now women). They are looking for careers that more successfully balance professional, family and social needs. Hospital medicine, with its reformed hours and increased numbers of consultant posts, has become steadily more attractive to the current crop of junior doctors. Paradoxically this has occurred at a time when many older consultants have become increasingly disillusioned with their lot – believing there has been a decline in power and status to fundholders, disliking the attentions of hospital management and its attendant erosion of clinical freedom, and believing the influx of additional posts will dilute the consultant's position, knowledge base and traditional role.

The recently introduced 'out of hours' scheme was a reflection of GPs' discontent, and at the time of writing its full effects have yet to be seen on clinical practice and referral rates.[42] Patient watchdog groups fear that the scheme (which provides funds for groups of practices to establish out of hours centres and ask patients to come to them rather than provide night visits (except for emergencies)) will reduce access to primary care. Those deemed particularly at risk are the elderly and the socially deprived as they are least likely to have access to transport. From one point of view the initiative brings British general practice closer to the norm in America where an out of hours visit from a primary care physician is rare. The neutral observer would be likely to regard this as a retrograde step – both in terms of access to services and the likely impact on secondary care through an increased propensity to refer/self-refer directly to hospital. It is too early to say whether this will occur in the UK, or whether the scheme will improve GP morale.

The 1990 GP contract remains widely disliked, principally because many GPs believe the remuneration remains too low and involves activities and paperwork to which they attach little value. In truth, the contractual relationship with what remains a group of self-employed businessmen is likely to remain a difficult issue. Yet the bottom line is that a failure to meet GP concerns, which would make the job more attractive (and also would require more resources), will lead to further recruitment and re-tention difficulties. The net result will be that primary care will be unable to fulfil its intended role. Yet if we are to understand the positions of the major political parties it is crucial to their plans that it does so.

Patients are becoming more assertive and litigious and tend to have less respect for the professional status of doctors. GPs feel themselves to be the meat in the sandwich between raised public expectations and what services are actually available. There is the widespread suspicion that both fundholding and the more nebulous 'GP commissioning' enables govern-ment and its agents – the civil service and health authorities – to distance themselves further from rationing issues, leaving doctors with the problem of deflecting their patients' demands. Bogle and Chisholm summarize the position thus:[43]

> This agenda of constant change and policies imposed on an unwilling profession has caused a sense of powerlessness, loss of independence, and demoralisation, which have contributed to increasing numbers of early retire-ments and a retirement crisis in general practice. By its actions, the govern-ment showed that it no longer valued its partnership with the profession.

The above makes for an inauspicious casting of primary care as the agent of change and the purchasing arm of the NHS. These weaknesses are com-pounded by the almost total absence of any training outside of the clinical arena for GPs. Successive Conservative administrations have never fleshed out their vision of a fundholding-led NHS but a moments reflection would lead the neutral observer to consider certain aspects of it somewhat biz-arre. Fundholding remains, operationally and philosophically, essentially a cottage industry – with accompanying disproportionate administrative costs – each practice pursuing its own course or working with others as it sees fit. It is assumed that the new health authorities will provide the organizational glue and supporting framework to ensure these doctors 'toe the line' but each party's roles and responsibilities remain unclear at the time of writing.

The NHS, meanwhile, continues to head towards a crisis in confidence as the gap between available resources and demand driven by demographics, technology and society's expectation widens. To this can be added the problems of a capital crunch, complicated by the uncertainties of obtaining purchaser support of schemes – where the 'purchaser' in effect may be dozens of fundholding practices.

Finally there is the paradox of GPs' motivation to become fundholders. This has already been alluded to in the breakdown of the 100 'representative' GPs. The logic of the Conservatives' approach – as publicly stated – is that fundholders will make the best purchasing decisions because they are closest to the patient and have first-hand knowledge of the clinicians who will undertake the treatments and the likely prognosis of each case. There is considerable merit in this approach which gives a sound reason for increasing the direct involvement of clinicians in both the purchasing and general decision-making process.

However, if the NHS is to operate effectively in anything like a market, those making the purchasing decisions (in this case doctors) must be prepared to respond to price/quality/access issues to force change. A failure to do so leaves the market stillborn. In effect, there must be a recognition that referral patterns might have to change. Ultimately, those providers found wanting should voluntarily or be forced to exit part or all of the market – particularly where there is over-supply relative to available resources (not to be confused with demand).

It is at this point that the fundholder's role becomes problematical. Many GPs become fundholders with two primary aims – to ensure the practice and its patients are getting the most out of the 'system' and to protect their local hospital. Local access naturally assumes a high priority. Most GPs are not nearly so concerned with ensuring macro-economic efficiency, ensuring supply meets available resources or even driving out poor-quality providers (particularly if it compromises the access issue).

These issues are better addressed at health authority level and there remains an expectation that these bodies will deliver these objectives. The means are now much less clear, however, whilst the potential for gridlock on contestable issues (for example closure of an accident and emergency department) are legion. Health authorities have traditionally found it difficult enough to deal with such issues in the past. They will now have to summon up the qualities of the Delphic Oracle on occasion. Their mandate has a less than solid foundation in any case when it is considered that the proposed shift is 'from Health Authorities purchasing with GP assistance to GP purchasing with Health Authority assistance' – a role somewhat akin to that of James Boswell to Dr Johnson, or perhaps Dr Watson to Sherlock Holmes.[44]

Where does this leave the internal market and more importantly the NHS? With a considerable number of unanswered questions and unfinished business. The public and many within the NHS may not care if the internal market withers away. What matters is if the issues the market (however inadequate) has helped to highlight – over-supply in certain areas, different costs, variable quality, well-off practices and poorly resourced ones – are ignored. The paradox is that in the USA, managed care organizations have the supporting infrastructure and techniques to facilitate these types of issues but no collective mandate to do so. The NHS has the mandate (otherwise why bother to have a national health service?) but seems to be intent in ensuring that the means are not in place to enforce it.

Furthermore there is the question of the sustainability of fundholding, given the resource and regulatory base that was established to encourage GPs to join the scheme.[45] In summary the concerns are as follows.

Practices are financed on the basis of historical referrals for the activities within the scheme. These historical expenditures become the basis for funding, without reference to list size, patient demographies or the host authorities' finances. Inadequacies in the original allocations or the pricing of elective activity affect all parties (fundholders and non-fundholders) as the pot of money available is fixed. Significantly the sum of these allocations as previously calculated (if all practices become fundholders) is likely to be greater than the health authority's actual resources (an example of the sum of the parts being greater than the whole)!

Budget-setting for a fundholding practice takes account of activity over a two-year period. During that time period non-recurring cash infusions are likely to have been made – waiting-list initiative (WLI) monies being the best-known example – allowing practices to purchase more activity (often at marginal rates). Yet the budgetary assessment takes into account all activity – however funded – thus creating two distortions. First, non-recurring activity/monies become recurring (and these practices also become eligible for any in-year non-recurring monies such as further WLIs (injections of monies by government with the aim of reducing waiting-lists and waiting times)). Second, historical volumes will be multiplied by the respective tariffs regardless of the price at which the volume is initially purchased. This problem is compounded by the fact that most hospitals do more cases in any one year than specified in their contracts. Payment for these cases is very likely to be at marginal rates at best ('free' cases are common). Next year's allocation will be based on last year's volume set at this year's full tariff (not marginal) price. From this it can be seen that disproportionately large sums will be taken from the remaining health authority contract.

Fundholding procedures are continually being extended and allocations adjusted accordingly. The new procedures tend to be much less frequent (most of the high-volume procedures were contained in the original scheme) increasing the chances of an abnormal allocation. This, in combination with the budget-setting requirements, increasingly leads to health authorities finding that the historical level of activity identified to fundholders is greater than the authority's total contract for the specialty in question!

Other inconsistencies include the system's failure to apply uniformly technical changes contained within the allocation letter, authority liability for fundholder overspends and cases exceeding a certain sum, an inconsistent funding base between waves of fundholders, the use of different currencies between fundholders and health authorities (chargeable procedures vs DRGs/HRGs cost and volume contracts etc.) – all of which should lead irresistibly to one conclusion. There has to be a rapid move to capitation-based funding.

Nearly everyone agrees with this – in principle. The problem is getting agreement to do something about it. Concerns are expressed about the fairness of various capitation formulae – as if policy-makers had suddenly discovered they should be concerned with equity, having previously pushed through a manifestly inequitable funding mechanism to establish the fundholding scheme. In truth these are smokescreens for the principal worry – that of rocking the boat. Capitation funding would create winners and losers and, as with the rest of the reforms, the problem is how to handle the losers. Furthermore, would extending the scheme to cover all GPs and all NHS activity, coupled with a reformed funding system, remove the very incentives to fundholding that drove the current enthusiasts to apply in the first place?

Rather than face these difficulties we are witnessing the behavioural characteristics of a corporate ostrich. However, these issues will not go away. Far from diminishing, they become more acute with each wave of fundholding. We could utilize the US capitation techniques previously described; the need is certainly there. Whether there is the will is another matter. Most of what has been written above holds true for the two alternative forms of GP purchasing – total fundholding and GP commissioning. Certainly the tension between any form of locality-based decision-making and the need for tight control on finances and policy will exist within any model likely to be seen in the UK. Whilst certain of the funding issues are particular to the way the fundholding scheme was established, the general issue of capitation vs historical activity funding has to be faced (even for 'shadow' budgeting) as does the question of incentives and deterrents.

Finally, this chapter would not be complete without an observation on two somewhat paradoxical situations. The first is on the current strong negotiating positions many fundholders enjoy relative to health authorities with providers. The second is the reluctance within the USA to embrace full capitation of physicians in a manner akin to fundholding. The situation with regard to the former would baffle many economists (at least those not conversant with the role politics plays in the NHS). The case against fundholding having any real negotiating power is made by Weiner and Ferris, and is in many respects the type of view likely to be held by Americans – whose market experience points firmly towards the 'God is on the side of the big battalions' theory of competition. The authors state: 'With the advent of open contracting by District Health Authorities which may be bargaining on behalf of upwards of a hundred thousand persons, it is not clear that a lone budget holding practice with 12,000 patients and no negotiating expertise will have much power. In the US, most successful managed care-hospital contracts involve far greater numbers ...'[22]

This view would be correct if DHAs were able to operate in a truly open contracting manner. However, this is not the case. During the annual contract negotiating process trusts typically have a predetermined income in mind, based essentially on them securing their centrally set financial targets – summarizable as a positive balance sheet and a 6% return on capital assets. Currently, the majority of that income has to come from health authorities. The greater the percentage (with one trust, my authority represented over 90% of their income), the greater the stakes – for both parties. The authority may be considered to be in a very strong position, until one realizes that there is an expectation that health authorities ensure that no trust within their particular geographic boundaries (which would normally be those for which it is the major purchaser) runs into undue financial difficulties.

This significantly changes the context of the negotiating process – particularly when chief executives and chairmen on either side of the table consider economic issues as subsidiary to 'wider' considerations. The screw is tightened by two further 'edicts' from above. The first is adherence to a predetermined timetable for getting such contracts agreed. Because of purchaser dependence on the timing of publication of the allocation letter (so as to ascertain what resources it has to start with), and the time it takes the finance department to clarify its technical content, negotiating time is very much at a premium.

The second is disapproval of 'rows in the NHS family' as manifested by a breakdown in negotiations and a need for 'external' arbitration.

Historically, considerable pressure has been put on both parties to avoid arbitration in Wales (there may be some variation in attitude elsewhere in the UK). Going to arbitration tends to be thought of as a career-threatening development, rather than a means of clarifying contractual issues and settling disputes that threaten to poison relationships for some considerable time.

The result can be poor contracts and, returning to our main theme, a focus on maximizing income from the principal purchasers (in contrast to many businesses which would discount steeply for big-volume purchasers and look to obtaining a more sizable profit at the margins). With the majority of its income secured, attention typically turns to the fundholders. In theory this contract process should have been running in parallel with the health authority negotiations, but often does not, for a number of reasons.

First, fundholders' allocations are normally finalized after the health authority monies are determined. Second, although in theory the same contracting timetable is applied to both health authorities and fundholders, in practice GPs are given more time. One reason is that fundholders when viewed as a series of individual practices are relatively small-scale purchasers and hence do not justify the attention of civil servants, etc. Another reason is that they are simply not as controllable as health authorities. There are many more fundholders than there are authorities and there is no direct line management relationship between a fundholder and the centre in the way there is, say between a health authority chairman and the secretary of state.

Third, fundholders often have a preference to negotiate low-volume contracts initially, with additional cases bought on a cost per case basis (if possible at marginal rates, although many trusts are countering this tactic by insisting that all volume up to last year's out-turn for the purchaser in question is set at full cost). Certain fundholders will also hang back as long as possible so as to 'shop around' for volume at marginal prices.

In response, trusts will probably wish to delay negotiating such contracts, until those with their principal purchasers are settled. Ideally, by that stage they have met their financial targets, or know the shortfall. Fundholder contracts can then be viewed essentially as 'marginal income'. Neither pricing nor timing differentials are supposed to occur, but are likely to remain a feature of NHS contracting as long as the following factors remain:

- health authorities remain the largest single purchaser of services for a trust
- the previously noted time lag remains in determining fundholder allocations

- fundholder resistance to regimentation and the desire of policy makers to keep doctors 'on board'

- the use of chargeable procedures as a separate contracting methodology for fundholders – making comparisons with health authority contracts on pricing issues difficult

- the inadequacy of external audit on trust pricing policies and the inability of heath authorities to enforce the normal leverage associated with being the major purchaser.

Eventually if all purchasing is undertaken by GPs these issues will no longer be relevant. No doubt they would be replaced by new problems as yet largely unidentified, or currently embryonic in character. Because of all governments' fear of alienating GPs, it may be that the UK is destined to have a two-tier purchasing environment which goes on for years, leaving in its wake chronic 'institutionalized' problems for health authorities (aka the perpetual funding crisis). Even if the funding distribution becomes entirely equitable between purchasing bodies, the tension with hospitals will remain (regardless of whether GPs or health authorities are leading the process of providing funds) if the secondary sector considers there are insufficient resources being made available for the services being demanded. Crucially, this issue remains constant, even if an internal market no longer exists.

Finally we return to the USA, and ask two interrelated questions: why global capitation for primary care physicians is not being introduced more quickly, and whether there are any markers for the UK in this. The reluctance to embrace full capitation has already been alluded to and broadly falls into the concerns listed below:

- doctors fear it will be ultimately used to drive their incomes down

- doctors and patient pressure groups are concerned that it will undermine the doctor–patient relationship

- it is not certain whether the situation will tend towards the idea that 'best care is no care', putting quality accordingly at risk. Capitation on its own rewards low-cost providers, whether of good or poor quality. To say that quality and cost-efficiency can move together is not to say that they will

- it is less than clear that markets can identify, much less penalize, poor clinical quality. The health care industry has had considerable problems documenting efficacy of work – either good or bad

- public policy issues must be considered – individual practitioners' decisions may conflict with wider public policy considerations. A hundred

different perspectives on health care do not readily translate into a coherent view on strategic issues – in the same way that the gross national
product of Denmark is not found by asking a statistically significant
random sample of people to have a stab at it

- physicians and practices have differing abilities to manage the finances
  of full capitation effectively. This is accompanied by concerns over
  training, support and accountability issues

- there is an overemphasis on financial and 'funding' issues (a price-
  driven, not quality-driven market).

Overall, these are familiar concerns expressed with regard to the fundholding scheme (particularly total fundholding), and some would also
impact on a GP commissioning model. All are legitimate issues which give
credence to the description of 'full personal capitation' and 'global capitation' as 'nuclear forces ... Highly, unarguably effective; hazardous in the
absence of strong controls'.[46] The message here is that such methods are
powerful, but potentially destructive.

This could be used to characterize total fundholding, even though it is
not necessarily funded by capitation or impacts directly on GPs' incomes.
On the latter issue, this is a mixed blessing for policy makers. On the one
hand, it reduces the chances of personal financial considerations intruding
on the clinical process – a major concern in the USA. On the other, it raises
questions about the incentive for changes in behaviour and the enthusiasm
for continuing when the going gets tough. Conventional wisdom in the
USA is that variable compensation must be in the 20–30% range (beyond
base) to capture attention and change performance. Variable compensation in the 5–15% range is considered 'completely wasted'.[46]

One can take issue with the percentages, but it does raise the broad
issue of remuneration of GPs for participating in the commissioning process. Currently, there is no direct relationship between personal income
and performance as a fundholder, which seems illogical. However if a link
is established, how much personal income should be 'at risk', and what
percentage variable for performance is desirable?

In the USA, capitation enthusiasts see the root cause of success coming
from the creation of a strong, direct tie between physicians' income and
the elimination of unnecessary care. Income levels can vary by more than
100%, depending on individual performance. In the UK the incentives are
likely to have to be more subtle and indirect. This makes the task more
difficult, and the warning in the US literature is ominous: devolving finances
to clinicians through capitation must 'not be implemented cavalierly –
precisely because full personal capitation [is] so effective in changing PCP

behaviour, [the] network bears "extra burden" of ensuring quality is not compromised ... Safeguards are necessary to minimize individual physicians' uncertainty, identify quickly potential lapses in judgement and ensure that such lapses do not recur'.[46]

The need for risk pools within fundholding, to help deal with unexpected cost volatility, has already been stated. It is worth noting that in the complete absence of stop-loss provisions US actuaries believe a minimum population of 25 000–50 000 (depending on its make up) is required to become actuarially stable.[46] Physician participation within a larger network helps to deal with this problem, but managed care companies fulfil a greater role than merely acting as a financial umbrella. 'Devolution' should not mean 'abdication'. There is an ongoing requirement for orientation, monitoring, information, advice, feedback, audit and the identification and resolution of inappropriate practices – all of which requires an adequate supporting infrastructure.

One reason why both HMOs and physicians sometimes hesitate to embrace full capitation, is because of their concerns about both parties' ability to fulfil these roles. Moreover, US contracting relationships (as previously explained) are usually complex affairs. A significant complicating factor is the existence of specialists operating separately from the hospitals. Separate contracts have to be placed with both parties (also remembering that each specialty is a separate contract), unless you can get one party (typically the hospital) to assume risk for the other – who then acts as a subcontractor. In contrast, NHS contracting is simpler and is likely to remain so.

In the UK the advent of total fundholding, with alliances of large practices producing covered populations of up to 100 000 persons, raises the stakes in the capitation game. By US standards, these are actuarially stable populations, whilst the organizational form is not dissimilar to an IPA. Are these set to become mini-health authorities (the term is used deliberately to imply a set of formal reporting and accounting relationships)? Large, collaborative total fundholding schemes raise a whole raft of interesting opportunities and issues of which the method of funding is but one more question. Essentially the same issues could be addressed at the rival model of GP Commissioning Groups. The only certainty appears to be that the NHS – like USA health care – continues to experience rapid change in its system of health care without much in the way of a blueprint to judge success or failure. In the case of the UK, this is particularly unacceptable, as unlike the USA, there is an explicit and legitimate expectation that government sets out the strategy, direction and structure of health care.

Conclusion

A strong case can be made for total fundholding being the natural body for purchasing within the NHS. If so, it should be based on a capitation model, with carrots and sticks at least at practice level (and possibly for the individual GP) for performance. There remain many unanswered (and perhaps unanswerable) questions concerning the role of the health authorities and their relationship with GPs as purchasers. These revolve around money (how to allocate it, and also dealing with over- and under-spends), quality (poor clinical performance, minimum standards in contracts, outcomes), information (who needs to see what, peer review, identification of outlier etc.), planning and priorities (implementation of national policy, formulation and implementation of plans, rationing, consultation on closures and general market management) and finally responsibilities – where will the buck stop?

One difficulty with all models of GP commissioning (especially total fundholding) is that the GP is both a purchaser and a provider. This creates opportunities for effective substitution of services by the practice, as it decides which things to provide 'in house' as opposed to being referred into secondary, community and social care. But the blurring of roles can also create problems as outlined with the US concerns with 'full capitation'. Taking this further, whatever the economic merits of 'owning' and running their own cottage hospitals and nursing homes, there are genuine conflicts of interest which may prove insurmountable for the UK public opinion.

There are many potential traps in this way forward. However, those opposed to such initiatives need to be aware that there is a vast difference between merely realizing that you dislike the direction health care reform is taking, and coming up with a sustainable, coherent, and financially realistic alternative. Those solutions that ignore the motivating forces of different contracting mechanisms, and rely on a combination of rhetoric and decree to drive change, will fail.

We have travelled some distance from this chapter's initial focus on reimbursement mechanisms. The somewhat dry subjects of risk pools and withholds may have been of interest to only a few readers. However, in contracting (as in much of medicine), the devil is in the detail. America, having never seemingly had a comprehensive national health care policy, periodically 'discovers' this, as its attack on one problem only creates others. Much of this chapter – and indeed the book as a whole – serves to demonstrate that they are no longer alone in this respect.

5

Quality and utilization review

I began asking Chicago area hospitals for their bypass mortality rates. I wasn't prepared for the responses I got. One hospital told me that I could get its mortality rate from the American Medical Association. Another said it didn't keep mortality rates. Yet another said I had no right to ask for such confidential information. All were falsehoods. Feeling desperate and at a disadvantage, I stooped to asking a friendly hospital secretary to get mortality rates for her facility during her off hours, when no one was around. A good thing I checked: patient outcomes there were poor ... There is something fundamentally wrong when a patient or a patient's family is made to feel like criminals simply for acting like sensible consumers.

Walt Bogdanich in *The Great White Lie*

The above eloquently sets out the case for the consumer, and unfortunately reflects the health industry's typical response to those demands. It is international in nature – substitute London, Bonn or New York for Chicago – and the relevance of the text remains. In the case of the UK the rise of consumerism is particularly troubling to an organizational ethic which has traded heavily on the idea of professional altruism towards a public which has a right to treatment but at the time, place and manner of the clinician's choosing. Patients were always patients and never customers. This is starting to change and the degree to which the 'internal market' promotes informed consumerism will be one measure of its success against its declared objectives.

A proper concern for quality and a desire to communicate the results of audit are long overdue in medicine. The former has a somewhat chequered history, the latter next to no history. There remains considerable opposition within health care to judging institutions and doctors on the quality of the care they provide and even more so to letting the results of such studies be known outside of self-selected circles.

Unsurprisingly, managed care companies are leading the way in terms of systematic quality review, and whilst that journey is by no means completed, best practice in the USA is some way in front of the UK. Moreover, US management and physicians are used to the idea of the patient as a customer. The challenge is to allow the consumer to make 'informed' choices. The UK mindset is much more resistant to this notion. Health authority officials charged with both involving clinicians in management and increasing clinical accountability will find managed care efforts in this area instructive.

Techniques apart, a cultural change in attitudes is required, involving primarily a willingness to question the actions of doctors and an over-arching concern for the well-being of the patient rather than the clinician, hospital, health authority, or the government of the day. It should be apparent that this applies as much (if not more so) to NHS management as it does to health professionals.

This is a tall order. Those wishing to change things could do with all the help they can get. This chapter highlights some key quality control techniques currently in use. One could easily write an entire book on quality issues in health care, but the focus of this section is primarily on the present use of quality monitoring and the management of utilization. If improvements can be made in these areas, we will have made significant progress in the quality arena.

Utilization review techniques

Utilization management can be defined as deliberate action to induce a more economical mix of treatment inputs without sacrificing health outcomes. This can take many forms, some of which currently receive scant attention in the UK. This is an area of managed care operations that may be seen as more easily transferable than any other, as the importance of the subject matter – the promotion of good quality, effective and efficient health care – is assisted by the relatively common approach to the delivery of medical care in the industrialized West.

However, utilization review remains a controversial area – particularly for clinicians, many of whom resent what they see as an expensive system for second-guessing their decisions, eroding clinical freedom and delivering substandard care. Part of this debate is engendered by the question of whether utilization review has at its heart a concern for simple cost-cutting, or whether the focus is on delivering the best and most appropriate care. Terms such as 'best' and 'appropriate' are themselves value-ridden but it has to be conceded that utilization review can be – and has been – abused on occasion. There is also the nagging doubt that whilst good quality care may often also be cost-effective care, there will be occasions that the 'appropriate' level of service may prove unaffordable. At its heart is a deep discomfort with the idea of putting monetary values on both the quality of life and life itself. Currently the talk is of a need to find more collaborative methods of managing quality and cost-effectiveness. This may help matters, but it is unlikely to eliminate the points of tension, representing as they do 'core' values for many health professionals. Clinicians typically make poor utilitarians.

Set out below are the principal tools in the inventory, and each has its advocates – receiving additional emphasis or falling out of favour on a regular basis. As a difficult area heavily laced with cynicism (on the motives of all the parties concerned), and inertia to change, the inclination to pass over quality issues is understandable. Despite regular proclamations to the contrary, it remains a marginal subject in the UK, where attention remains focused on numbers – of those treated and still waiting to be treated.

In the USA the different emphasis can be illustrated from this quote in Weiner and Ferris:[22]

> From the start of the HMO movement, quality was *the* preeminent issue. Detractors vehemently believed that the financial and organisational structure of HMOs were incompatible with good care. Supporters, just as vehemently believed it was the HMO concept that led to good care.

In this atmosphere, combined with the attentions of the most litigious society in history, can be found useful techniques and systems that will help give the subject the attention it deserves within the NHS.

Provider selection

One of the most effective ways to ensure proper utilization is to select those doctors with a track record of efficient practice and then induce preferential use of these clinicians. Some managed care organizations make significant use of this method of utilization management – unlike in the UK. Significantly, this technique has seen little use in the approval of fundholding applications by practices, or in medical audit, and one may hypothesize that the reasons for this are due to some or all of the following:

- the Conservative government wished both to promote the concept of fundholding and increase the absolute numbers of fundholding GPs. In pursuit of this it generally looked to liberalize the selection process rather than introducing more rigorous acceptance criteria (the same kind of dynamics tends to apply when managed care companies are keen to expand their physician network)

- the scheme's construction is built around an ability to record clinical activity (during the preparation year) and not the clinical validity of the activity itself

- there remains an expectation that the health authority will act as the pressure valve and 'bank of last resort' for fundholders

- the conventional wisdom is that there are inadequate data to allow conclusions to be drawn as to who are the efficient GPs (or, more to the point, the inefficient ones). Moreover, there was little tradition, capacity or inclination amongst FHSAs to engage in such a debate even if such information had been available. The new authorities have yet to show that they are prepared to be more proactive in this area

- general practice has a tradition of operating voluntary disclosures of information and voluntary participation in audit only. In such an environment it is unsurprising that both data and participants may be incomplete.

In the newly constituted health authorities the subject of provider selection and retention is likely to gain in emphasis – if only in response to the increasing sums of public money being devolved directly to GPs. This is a difficult area, often requiring diplomacy and tact, but it is one that has to be addressed. Boland quotes one national preferred provider organization (PPO) manager as estimating that the exclusion of inefficient physicians, via analysis of claims data, reduced annual per enrollee health care costs by about 10%.[47] In the US poor physician selection is likely to be a substantial contributor to a plan not making budget or even to its ultimate failure.

Unsurprisingly, a major problem, even in the USA, is obtaining meaningful information about individual performance. Even when available it may be considered too expensive to obtain and review, and the results too problematic to act upon. In such an environment it makes considerable sense to designate provisional status to those physicians joining a plan so as to facilitate postselection management of practice habits and if necessary their deselection.

As a unitary organization the NHS has the advantage of theoretically being much better placed than the average managed care company for devising the required data sets, collecting and analysing them and ultimately selecting and regulating doctors in this context. More effective provider selection might largely negate the need for some of the expensive and time-consuming utilization review techniques discussed below, by tackling the issue at the 'front door' rather than trying to pick up the pieces after the event.

How many 'bad doctors' are there? The term itself would need careful
definition, particularly with regard to utilization issues where an inability
to work within a predefined budget would be regarded by many as hardly
a good reason for being marked as a 'bad doctor'. (In fact an almost complete disregard for the financial consequences of a clinical course of action
is seen by some clinicians and members of the public as a prerequisite of
being a 'good doctor'.) *Medical Economics* in January 1992 reported that
in the USA only one doctor in 400 receives a suspension, revocation or
gets put on probation per annum.[48] It concluded that the number which
should be cited was nearer 2% or eight times the current incidence of
official action taken. This, coupled with the concerns of bodies as diverse
as Illiych and an examination by the Royal College of Surgeons into perioperative deaths to the widely reported variations in patient referrals, costs
and outcomes can only lead to a conclusion that organizations need to display greater diligence with regard to their initial selection of clinicians.[49,50]

Provider education

Educating doctors in the most cost-effective treatments and prompting the
use of evidence-based medicine represents another avenue of utilization
management. This area, which should also include medical/clinical audit,
has a longer tradition on both sides of the Atlantic and has generated
a considerable amount of literature. However, the ability of education –
on its own – to modify behaviour positively remains equivocable at best.
Traditionally, doctors have been largely ignorant of the costs of medical
care – and perhaps more surprisingly of the effectiveness of many diagnostic and treatment regimens. Awareness of costs and a drive towards
outcomes-based medicine can be observed in both countries, but there
remains a considerable way to go, with progress being at best modest in
both areas. The use of education on cost-containment issues and medical
audit programmes for all levels of the medical hierarchy (in both countries)
are attended by considerable scepticism as to their effectiveness – particularly over anything other than the short term. The use of education alone
appeals to many practitioners and teachers alike as befitting the rational/
intellectual paradigm medicine likes to think it occupies. Moreover, the
non-coercive overtones suits a profession jealous of its autonomy. The
unfortunate reality seems to be that to extend its effectiveness beyond
the temporary arena requires a continuing programme, administrative
support and (most important of all from the standpoint of this book) direct and indirect economic incentives. As Boland observes: 'Newly learned
behaviour requires reinforcement or it will die out.'[47]

It is the degree to which managed care organizations attempt to complement education with other levers to modify behaviour that is of interest here. As previously noted, US observers tend towards the view that economic incentives are a powerful tool for reducing unnecessary utilization, but these have to be of sufficient size to act as meaningful motivators. The whole issue of financial rewards and penalties is controversial. There is little consensus that such methods work, and even less on whether they are ethical. The author believes that there is sufficient anecdotal evidence to conclude that doctors will respond to economic incentives if they are:

• well constructed

• large enough to get and retain attention

• directly related to a doctor's own behaviour.

As a tool, they can be used for both ethical and unethical purposes, and should be judged in the light of the intentions of those proposing change, rather than the tool itself.

The utilization review process

Traditionally, the utilization review (UR) process has been the principal platform by which managed care has attempted to control medical and utilization-related costs. The development of capitation-based risk models may serve to reduce UR's importance internally, but it is probably more realistic to see such models as complementary tools rather than direct replacements for UR.

The UR department will typically follow Sutton's law and focus on 'where the money is'. Traditionally, this means that most attention is given to inpatients, and encompasses preservice, concurrent and retrospective review, second opinion management and specific case management. In contrast, the utilization review function within NHS purchasing is skeletal. What is not being proposed here is the creation of mirror images of an HMO's medical care management structure, as this is both unaffordable and largely unnecessary. However, there are some processes of interest, and these could be applied selectively.

Authorization systems

The presence of an authorization system could be said to be one of the defining elements of managed health care. The first requirement in an authorization system is to define what does and does not require authorization. This is tied to the various benefit packages members have and therefore it is important members and providers are aware of the authorization process. There is probably no plan that requires authorization of all services – for instance, before seeing a primary care physician – but typically services not provided by the PCP will require some form of authorization (referral to a specialist, diagnostic services, hospitalization and surgical procedures). However, more liberal plans – such as PPO indemnity – will typically be less stringent in these matters. The rule of thumb is that the tighter the authorization system, the greater the plan's ability to manage utilization.

Authorization has three main objectives:

• to ensure the proposed clinical intervention is covered by that particular member's benefit plan (see Appendix IV for examples of 'evidence of coverage' in plans. These detail typical exclusions)

• to ensure that where a protocol for the management of a particular condition exists it is being followed

• in the case of inpatient and expensive treatment, to forewarn the medical care management department that a patient is entering hospital so that they can be appropriately treated and reviewed, and discharge planning can commence. In the case of particularly high-risk/expensive cases, individual case management may well be provided.

All three objectives highlight the proactive nature of medical care management, although of course in the real world there are many occasions when a member is unable to obtain prior authorization, e.g. emergency admissions, urgent problem occurring out of area.

The protocols used will normally include clinical criteria that have to be met before the intervention in question is considered, perhaps where the intervention must take place (e.g. at a certain hospital, as a day case) and what pretreatment tests can be provided, where and when. If the provider fails to follow these protocols, the claim is likely to be refused or only paid in part.

Sentara has around 180 authorization protocols (see Appendix V for some generic examples). Despite the number of protocols, UK readers may be surprised to find that among the hospital procedures which did not require any pre-authorization were requests from PCPs for magnetic resonance imaging (MRI) and computed tomography (CT) scans.

What makes for successful UR? Boland considers that there are in essence six components found in effective UR programmes:[47]

- reviewer knowledge. UR programmes generally rely on nurses as the frontline reviewers. Questionable cases are typically referred on to the medical director's physician team. As can be seen from the authorization protocols in Appendix V, an experienced reviewer is required if the 'protocols' are not going to be seen as so vague that they are effectively ignored

- reviewer courage. Because UR is seen by many doctors as an unjustified attack on their clinical freedom, the process has an inherent level of 'measured confrontation' if it is to be meaningful. As a result, 'burn out' is always a potential problem, and it is essential that reviewers obtain consistent support from senior management if disillusionment is not quickly to set in

- system integrity. To work effectively, the UR must be free of major loopholes. To put it bluntly, if doctors can easily get round the authorization process by a mixture of exaggeration and guile, its value will be compromised

- the quality and rigour of standards. UR programmes are by no means uniform in the USA, and this is reflected in key performance indicators such as hospital days per 1000 members which vary from less than 200 to over 700. Sentara, which probably runs a fairly 'liberal' scheme (by West Coast standards), refuses around 2% of authorization requests on benefit and medical necessity grounds (around 800 cases per annum). This has a significant administrative impact given that contested denials can go to peer review and appeals committee

- the attitude of the medical community is self-explanatory. The degree of hostility or acceptance to UR will be influenced in a number of ways – the quality and personability of reviewers, the rigorousness with which the provider network has been chosen, ongoing education, the amount of time UR takes for the physician and his staff, etc.

- benefits design and the ability of the system to leverage good quality care. An example might be delays in discharge because home health benefits are not covered, or the provision of a piece of medical equipment to allow the patient to be treated at home.

To the above should be added the complementary (or otherwise) impact on the reimbursement and risk models in place with providers.

Control methods

In addition to the above, the following UR controls may be in place:

- single-visit authorization only (with the normal exceptions – chemotherapy, obstetrics, mental health, physical therapy)

- refusal to pay member claims where authorization process has not been followed, e.g. self-referral to the accident and emergency department for a minor injury/illness

- prohibition of secondary referrals by consultants without PCP/UR authorization

- assignment of maximum allowable length of stay – this is based on the admission diagnosis and gives a target for both discharge planning and claims processing. This is often associated with a per diem based contract with plans refusing to pay beyond the maximum length of stay amount

- compulsory obtainment of a second opinion for a proposed intervention

- retrospective analysis of multipatient data to establish trends – showing doctors how their practice compares with average patterns for a geographic area and/or specialty is generally thought to be one of the more influential ways of changing practice (as is medical record review)

- influencing members – use of copayments, the authorization process and PCPs acting as gatekeepers.

UR for many remains a policing action – in mindset and execution. The introduction of capitation is leading to changes in UR's traditional role, with physicians increasingly seeing it as a supporting process to help them prosper in the 'new world' and will hopefully become philosophically integrated over time with the wider quality arena. The current enthusiasm in the UK for clinical effectiveness/evidence-based purchasing as a collaborative programme directed by clinicians and emphasizing collaborative working is a welcome development. However, it has to be underpinned by a determination to monitor performance and make changes when problems are noted. Achieving a balance between overreliance on persuasion vs coercion, and providing a means of support vs the creation of bureaucratic controls, is clearly difficult.

Moving forward on quality issues

There are many different definitions of quality. A common approach is to accept that quality has a dual meaning. First, quality refers to freedom from errors or deficiencies (a zero error rate). Second, quality refers to product features that meet certain customer needs and thereby provide customer satisfaction. In the realm of health care, it seems both uncontroversial and common sense to assert that it is essential that measurements verify that providers are delivering appropriate care and achieving favourable outcomes, but there is surprisingly little activity taking place on these subjects.

The reasons for this are many, amongst them being a lack of conventions and methods for assessing health care quality. In an area of operations which is often considered to be labour-intensive and subjective to the point of trying to nail blancmange to the ceiling, NHS purchasers have generally concentrated their efforts on price and volume issues and left quality to the nurses and sociologists. Although at one level this is entirely understandable (given the pressures in these areas generated by ministerial/ civil servant attention), it also lays the NHS open to the charge that it is customer-oriented in the same way that a sausage factory is pig-oriented.

The USA's performance on monitoring and acting upon quality indicators is, like much else, a mixed bag. Its fundamental weakness – as a health system – is its fragmented structure. For example, any large-scale longitudinal study is hampered by the multitude of insurers and plans. They in turn may use different definitions, and patients may move plans and companies. So, for example, the question 'do people who enrol in plan A experience better outcomes in heart surgery than plan B or no plan at all?' is likely to elicit the answer: 'Don't know'. Plan A has only been around for 'x' years and was restructured in 1991, changing its member base, whilst plan B has a different population mix!

However, quantifiable information about the quality of health care has become an important issue for employer groups and part of the industry's response has been to develop the Health Plan Employer Data and Information Set (HEDIS). HEDIS was developed by the National Committee for Quality Assurance (NCQA) in conjunction with a coalition of health insurers and major employers. Its aim is to create a standardized, consistent and objective method for defining health care value and to develop the tools necessary to measure that value. The emphasis, therefore, is the use of standardized definitions and methodologies for obtaining performance measures from each health plan and uniform presentation of the information.

There are elements of HEDIS that open up opportunities for international comparisons (international collaboration on quality issues has considerable potential). HEDIS attempts to present a 'snapshot' of four areas:

- quality of care

- member access and satisfaction

- membership and utilization

- finance.

Not all these areas are suitable or relevant for transatlantic comparison, but elements of quality of care, member access and satisfaction, and utilization should be of interest.

Quality of care encompasses:

- childhood immunization (by vaccine)

- cholesterol screening

- mammography screening

- cervical cancer screening

- low birthweight and prenatal care measures

- asthma inpatient admissions and readmissions

- outpatient follow up after hospitalization for a mental disorder

- diabetic retinal examination.

Member access and satisfaction includes:

- the percentage of members with at least one visit to a plan physician in the previous three years

- waiting time for non-urgent, symptomatic office visit (general and mental health), target and actual

- waiting time for urgent, symptomatic office visit (general and mental health), target and actual

- waiting time for emergency care (general and mental health), target and actual

- member satisfaction (with plan, PCPs, competence of PCP etc.).

Utilization includes:

- high occurrence/high-cost DRGs – discharges per 1000; average cost per discharge, average length of stay

- frequency of selected procedures – male and female (e.g. cardiac catheterization, coronary artery bypass graft (CABG), angioplasty, cholecystectomy, laminectomy and prostatectomy

- inpatient admissions per 1000 – total acute medicine/surgery, maternity, neurology

- inpatient days per 1000 – total acute medicine/surgery, maternity, neurology

- average length of stay – total acute medicine/surgery, maternity, neurology

– note: all of the above broken down by age groups

- outpatients – total visits – visits per 1000

- emergency room – total visits – visits per 1000

- day cases – total visits – visits per 1000

– note: all of the above broken down by age groups

- inpatient utilization – non-acute care (excluding mental health and chemical dependency)

- measures by age group for the following categories: admits, days, admits per 1000, days per 1000, average length of stay

- mental health – inpatient discharges and average length of stay by age and gender (including per 1000)

- mental health utilization: percentage of members receiving services – inpatient/outpatient (by age and gender)

- readmissions for mental health disorders – age, gender, members hospitalized, percentage readmitted within 90 and within 365 days

- same measures as above for chemical dependency

- outpatient drug utilization by age group – average cost of prescriptions PMPM – average number of prescriptions PMPM.

Some of these measures can be found in the UK; others (for instance the use of rates per 1000 and procedure-specific analysis), although not new, are not given the same exposure or attention. As discussed in the next chapter, the rate per 1000 measure is a particularly illuminating report, and could usefully be adopted within the NHS, where so much attention has been given to activity and reducing waiting-lists that the crucial question of treatment rates has tended to be overlooked.

Within the contract itself, quality issues may seem conspicuous by the scarcity of reference to them (Appendix I). The provider may only be required to submit materials which demonstrate an active quality assurance programme as delineated by the Joint Commission on Accreditation of Healthcare Organisations (JCAHO). This is a deceptively simple request, as obtaining JCAHO (and other recognized accreditating organizations in the USA) accreditation is far from easy. US observers familiar with NHS hospitals doubt whether many or any at all could pass JCAHO standards.

Quality indicators that might well be required for submission include:

- patient satisfaction

- adjusted mortality rates within 30 days of hospitalization for the 20 most frequently performed procedures

- number of readmissions within two weeks of discharge related to the last admission

- number of unplanned returns to the operating room for complications related to a previous surgical procedure during current admission

- nosocomial infection rates based on infections which first become apparent 72 or more hours after admission

- number of adverse drug reactions or medication errors with serious potential for harm

- number of unexpected deaths

- details of any untoward incidents including actions taken.

If the NHS is to move to an accreditation-based approach to quality issues, it needs to recognize that many UK providers would fall some way short of North American standards. If the process is to have any meaning, it has to be both rigorous and systematic.

Conclusion

As has been previously noted medical management is the very essence of managed care. This has required HMOs to develop and maintain relationships with providers and practitioners, negotiate with them, and educate them. Managing an efficient provider network is crucial to cost-containment and the marketability of managed care. This puts a premium on the skills of negotiation, persuasion, analysis and a willingness and ability to communicate medical management issues to doctors. Health authorities in their new role have essentially the same agenda and skills requirement. As has been previously noted, the experience of HMOs is particularly relevant in the medical management arena. One area in which HMOs are typically better than the NHS is engaging clinicians in a systematic process of analysis and discussion on performance issues. They have a powerful incentive, money; but equally important is their individual, practice and plan reporting capability and their willingness to use it. In this arena the average US company operates from a weaker position than the health authorities. Typically the managed care company's patients will only represent a percentage of the physician's total business and this has a direct impact on the HMO's associated leverage. Computerized links with practices and the use of dedicated executive information systems (EIS) or decision support systems (DDS) are relatively rare. Comparative data (beyond the company) can be difficult to find and/or present. Health authorities, in contrast, could make use of all these advantages but typically fail to do so.

NHS management must be prepared to change its mindset with regard to medical management issues. Regular comparative performance reports must become the norm. Above all, these must be distributed to, and discussed with, clinicians. Physician profiles should be constructed based on utilization reviews to analyse practice habits (for example a tendency to overrefer or underrefer to consultants), outcomes measurement and patient satisfaction surveys.

Alongside changes to attitude is an absolute requirement to improve the flow of information. This is common both to devolved and centralized models of health care and quality management. The information deficit and some possible remedies are considered in the next chapter.

6

Management information systems

It should be apparent from what has already been written that managed care is an information-dependent process. An HMO that is not investing adequately in its MIS infrastructure is like a battleship which has substandard electronic weapons and control systems. It may look impressive on the outside, but when it comes to the test of battle it will perform inadequately compared with its more modern counterparts.

The American health care industry recognizes the importance of its MIS environment to current operations and future prosperity. Investment issues relating to MIS are typically one of the key strategic issues for a company. As a result, there is an absence of the somewhat tedious questioning of the value of IT that continues to pervade the NHS. There remains the issue of those US executives and clinicians who can operate in an information-driven management system and those who feel threatened by it. However, few in either group would be comfortable declaring that such an infrastructure is of little relevance to their decision-making processes.

The MIS director in a typical US health care company is in an environment that is satisfying and yet frustrating at the same time: satisfying, because investment is usually a given, information is in great demand, and the complexity of the issues promotes security of employment, status and a comfortable salary; frustrating, because MIS systems in the USA often mirror their parent health system – fragmented, complex, and expensive to operate. The primary MIS challenge in the USA is the drive for integration and rationalization of systems. Alongside this is the need to develop true EIS. A major obstacle for an MIS strategy is how to integrate primary care physicians' office technology into that of the managed care company. The difficulty is that for many physicians the company in question will represent only a percentage of its total patient base. At its most basic, physicians do not want to integrate their systems with multiple payers (as this is technically and operationally complex, as well as being costly), but they are also typically reluctant to 'climb into bed' with a single payer. In contrast, the job of NHS technologists looks much simpler, although they in turn face other obstacles (resource constraints, getting uniform policies agreed, etc.) which may turn out to be at least as difficult to overcome.

Before consideration is given to the typical range of reports which an MIS is expected to provide, it is worth considering the relative state of IT investment, and the use made of it, between the two countries. As far as the NHS is concerned, investment in IT is noticeable by its absence of late. As recently as November 1995 the *Health Service Journal* described the hospital systems market as 'largely moribund because of tough controls on spending'.[51] Central monies have dried up and trusts find it hard to get purchaser support for any increase in costs related to IT investment (such incentives never seem to lead to lower costs). A recent paper by Locke concluded that published evidence on the value of IT to hospitals was 'scarce and far from conclusive'.[52]

The Achilles' heel of the IT business case – showing cash-releasing benefits – has taken on a new importance with the increasing reliance on private sector financing (Chapter 7). That there is an acute awareness of IT costs is unsurprising, the more puzzling issue being why it has proved so difficult to justify such investment in terms of conferring a business advantage which can be exploited in the market. Nowhere has this been more apparent than with the hospital information support systems (HISS) sites, once the proud flagships of the Resource Management Initiative.[33] Far from dominating the acute sector's IT environment (as both policy makers and computer suppliers hoped) they are struggling to convince a still sceptical service – and Treasury – that they are anything other than white elephants. Their basic problem is that currently NHS hospitals do not need such sophisticated MIS environments to operate successfully within the purchaser/provider system.

Paradoxically, the direct role of government and its agents – which in theory should have had the effect of promoting IT-related expenditure – has had a distorting and sometimes directly negative impact in IT in the NHS. This paradox has expressed itself in three ways:

The first is the pattern of MIS funding by government (either directly, e.g. Department of Health or Welsh Office, or indirectly through health authorities). The two most striking features of this are:

- an inequitable distribution of funding

- the high 'failure' rate of IT projects, particularly when measured against initial expectations.

The inequitable funding of IT is quite extraordinary for an organization which propounds equity as being one of its central values. Yet, some trusts have had capital investment in excess of ten million pounds whilst others have had to make do with less than 5% of that amount. These same agencies – who were supposed to be preparing all parties for the internal market – were also responsible for ensuring they operated from a level playing field. Is this due to conspiracy or cock-up? The author contends the latter. Those charged with formulating then implementing the IT strategy miscalculated its costs and timescales. Quite simply, they took too long and found that the earmarked monies would neither cover all the sites nor be rolled over by the treasury year after year as initial procurement and subsequent roll-outs dragged on interminably.

This brings us to the second area of government – or more accurately central bureaucracy's – negative influence. Their impact on IT procurement has been such that the process has become an end in itself. Given the possible embarrassment if flaws are subsequently discovered or a legal challenge is made, the pressures to run things by the (lawyer's) book has become all pervading. All too often the result can be characterized by the phrase 'perfect procurement, shame about the result'.

The need to follow a textbook procurement process illustrates the risk-adverse environment in which NHS management operates. Unfortunately such procurements – although technically flawless – all too often end up with the primary objective (for the user, at any rate) not being achieved. The objective is a system meeting user expectations, delivering the outcomes expected, at the right time and price. Yet a European Community (EC) Procurement (a formal, compulsory process to be followed by government agencies for member countries when procuring most goods and services) seems a plodding, adversarial process. Can it be different? Perhaps, but only when senior managers get serious about the use of MIS and assert themselves more over the process: because they, not the legal advisors, procurement managers or IT specialists, are the customer. Central funding has diluted this further because suppliers are encouraged to regard the bureaucracy allocating the funds (and often controlling the procurement process) as the customer.

The third area is the failure of government to create sufficient incentives within the NHS to utilize its MIS investment fully. This may seem a particularly contentious statement given the recent health service reforms, but the key words are 'sufficient' and 'fully'. The internal market has promoted the importance of previously rather unsung processes such as clinical coding, a good medical records system, and keeping one's patient administration system up to date. Improvements in these areas have in many places been dramatic and are not to be decried – nor should the abysmal starting point from which gains have been made be forgotten.

Nevertheless, the typical NHS purchaser or provider has yet to realize the potential of IT as a means of reengineering their respective organizations. The NHS is getting better at using IT to allow it to carry out basic organizational functions, i.e. count how many patients came through the door, run an appointments system, and analyse the workload of certain members of staff and departments. What is still too rarely seen is the use of IT to make radical changes in work practices, break down compartmentalization, make services more consumer-friendly, etc. All too often it seems to have the opposite effect with the various departments (pathology, radiology, records, finance etc.) each having their own departmental system aimed at automating existing practices.

Whilst acknowledging genuine advances, it has to be recognized that progress in the UK has not been uniform. Many boards, even when agreeing to IT investments, seem to do so with reluctance. Government has not done the computer industry any favours by seeming to confirm the view of the sceptics that decent information systems are a luxury, not a necessity. The best example of this is the production of contract minimum data sets. This should be the health service's equivalent of an invoice for services rendered. As can be seen from both physician and hospital contracts in the USA (outlined in the appendices) a failure to produce an itemized bill means no payment. In the NHS this most elementary example of normal business practice and information exchange has yet to be viewed as standard practice in an internal market that is supposed to have been operating for over five years!

The growth of fundholding and pressure from health authorities are finally leading to progress in this area. However, listed below are a number of provider responses the author encountered as recently as the 1994/5 contract round when requesting contract minimum data sets (CMDS):

- 'I don't see why you need them, don't you trust us?'

- 'We can't produce them until our new PAS is commissioned'

- 'We can give you the information but it will cost us money so we'll have to bill you.'

We return to the initial assertion that government has failed to create sufficient incentives within the NHS to utilize IT fully. The reforms have created trusts, established fundholding and looked to introduce a market economy to NHS affairs, but expediency has been allowed to override the requirement that a supporting infrastructure be created to facilitate such activities in advance, or at least in parallel to the reforms themselves. Hence some hospitals were approved for self-governing trust status with only the most rudimentary information capabilities – witness their consistent failure to produce CMDS. How long would a commercial enterprise survive if it were unable to raise invoices and track its own production?

This is the biggest single difference between the two health systems in their use of, attitude to and expenditure on IT. Health care organizations in the USA have yet to realize fully the liberating potential of the computer, but they do realize its vital role in day-to-day operations. No invoice, no payment. Payment itself is based on contracting methodologies – DRGs, per diems, discounted charges – that require information systems to process and report on them. The struggling IT suppliers to the NHS had better hope these practices are mandated in the near future. In one sense the firms serving the NHS have been victims of the muddle-headed decision to define the IT infrastructure before establishing the system within which it would operate – and be asked to pay its way.

By contrast, US systems are products of their environment and mirror its shortcomings. As previously noted, their historical development lies in the requirement to accurately record, bill and report on patient activity. Using an MIS as a means of integrating the disparate provider network, and gaining associated leverage from rationalization of the many systems in use, has only recently been on the agenda. Increasingly, managed care companies and others have 'discovered' the benefits of a coordinated approach to the delivery of care. As health care in the USA moves gradually into this new phase the advantage will go to those companies which have the imagination (and resources) to turn system integration into a reality and make use of modern communication facilities – the internet, electronic links etc.

The rest of this chapter looks at some standard reporting sets used in managed care and highlights those of potential interest to NHS purchasers. In reporting there is always a constant battle between the desire to pick up trends and adverse events early and being swamped with data masquerading as information. This problem transcends national borders and industries. A decent MIS should allow users the flexibility to choose which reports they want as routine and those required only on an ad hoc basis (without the need for expert intervention). The issue then becomes what should be routinely produced, and what triggers an ad hoc report.

A managed care company's reporting capability is likely to have three principal levels of focus. The first is a high-level view of company operations as a whole, which in turn will consist of an overview of each 'plan' (in Sentara's case, for example, Optima and SHP). This is the standard senior management/board reporting set. The second level will be the detail behind a particular set of operations (for example the performance by specialty). The third is individual doctor/practice utilization and cost reports. Most of these data originate from the claims process (the NHS equivalent of the CMDS) and are the building-blocks from which all three levels of reporting are essentially derived. The first point to be made in connection with the above is deceptively straightforward – that an NHS purchaser must also have this level of reporting capability. The traditional difficulty has been the production of practice-/doctor-level reports, for peer-group comparisons. To this can now be added a further dimension – the promotion of GP-led commissioning. If GPs are genuinely to assume the lead role they are likely to require both new and additional information reports and support. The issues this presents both health authorities and GPs have barely been touched upon at the time of writing. Many promoting this organizational form made a prior assumption that the supporting infrastructure exists, or is not an issue. They are wrong on both counts.

Board level key indicators

For a commercial enterprise, key indicators will include financial measures such as liquidity ratios, quick ratios and equity financing ratios that need not detain UK readers. However, their activity and budget reports are relevant. Of particular interest in a 'high-level report' might be the following:

- general reporting convention

- rate yield PMPM

- medical expense ratio

- hospital activity and expenditures PMPM.

General reporting convention

A subject is likely be reported on in terms of budgeted and actual expenditure for the current year and the previous financial year, plus for the two financial years in question: a current month and year to date analysis.

This facilitates an 'at a glance' appreciation of trends. It is surprising how often the question 'how were we doing this time last year' is not asked within the NHS because in part the information is not readily available. One objection the finance department may have to producing reports in such a format (apart from the work involved) is that 'too much has changed since last year' or even 'it isn't going to be relevant as we've merged with Authority X'. Neither is a good enough reason. If things have changed this can be explained when looking at the figures (perhaps things have not changed as much as one hoped). On the issue of authority amalgamation the need to amend reports to show historical activity both separately and as an amalgam of organizations is vital – otherwise the new organization has no 'corporate experience' on which to judge current events.

Rate yield PMPM

This is a standard performance measure. It shows what the average monthly premium is per member, with the actual value shown against budget, etc. This measure may not seem relevant to the UK but surely it would be a good idea to show the authority's allocation as an amount per resident? The 'budget' figure could be the finance director's initial estimate of this year's allocation. Moreover the same device could be used to show fundholding practices' allocations as an amount per patient on their list. This may well reveal interesting variations between practices.

Medical expense ratio

This is expressed as a percentage of total expenditure and reflects the amount actually spent on health services. In effect health authorities already produce such a figure as a derivative of the target for administrative costs. It may prove increasingly useful as an indicator of any creeping administrative, legal and miscellaneous costs in relation to fundholding as well as health authority expenditure.

Hospital activity and expenditures PMPM

What is of interest here is the very different reports a US company will produce under this heading compared with a health authority. The NHS reports are likely to focus on activity against target for each hospital it contracts with, costs against target for each contract and waiting-lists (again against each hospital). These are all essential reports. One is unlikely to see them in the USA – at least not as senior management reports. Waiting-lists are unlikely to be relevant but the omission of the other reports is less easy to explain (although hospitals are not often set predetermined activity levels). To the degree that there is a logical answer it lies in what does get reported.

The plan

The focus is on the performance of the plan as a whole and there are a number of standard reports to help highlight this. It is common for most plans to use bed days per 1000 plan members as a key measure. This is a very useful indicator, although rarely used in the UK. Defining what should count as a bed day is important. The following 'breakouts' for separate reporting are suggested for those interested in using this measure:

- exclude day cases

- decide whether to include nursery days for newborn infants when the mother is in hospital

- report geriatrics and psychiatry separately.

The use of bed days per 1000 is an excellent indicator of overall utilization, particularly when seen in association with the other reports described below. In the NHS attention has been focused for some time on activity and waiting-lists but this report alongside the admissions per 1000 and day cases and outpatient attendances per 1000 give a new dimension – is the population receiving more or less treatment in comparison with other areas and previous years? Further analysis by specialty, practice and emergency and elective caseload is likely to be illuminating.

A typical high-level managed care reporting set would have the following contents:

PMPM	Actual	Budget	Month	YTD	Yr 1	Yr 2
Inpatient cost/day						
Inpatient days of care/1000						
Inpatient cost/case						
Inpatient admissions/1000						
ALOS						
Average day-case cost						
Day cases/1000						

Because some of these are rarely used in the NHS but could be profitably exploited, some of the more complex formulae are given below.

Inpatient cost per day

With the proviso over what is included in the term 'inpatient' this should be a straightforward equation. This report could be run both at 'hospital' and 'all contracts' level. The former is probably the more common but the latter provides 'the big picture'.

Inpatient days of care per 1000

The standard formula is relatively straightforward. It can be used to calculate the annualized bed days per 1000 for any time period chosen (e.g. for the day, month to date, year to date etc.). Assume a 365-day year as opposed to a 12-month year to avoid variations due solely to the length of the month. The formula is as follows:

$$[A \div (B \div 365)] \div (C \div 1000)$$

where A is gross bed days per time unit, B is days per time unit and C is plan membership. Set out below is an example of the calculation for the month to date as it might apply to a health authority (substitute resident population for plan membership):

Assume:	Total gross hospital days in month to date (MTD)	= 4000
	Resident population	= 220 000
	Days in MTD	= 28
Step 1:	Gross days MTD	= 4000 ÷ (28 ÷ 365)
		= 4000 ÷ 0.0767
		= 52 151
Step 2:	Days per 1000 in	= 52 151 ÷ (220 000 ÷ 1000)
	MTD	= 52 151 ÷ 220
		= 237.05.

Therefore days/1000 for MTD = 237.

Inpatient cost per case

Like inpatient cost per day this is a simple equation which when set against a budget forecast and previous years, gives the board an immediate sense of the dynamics of patient care for the area in question.

Inpatient admissions per 1000

This indicator may help authorities to explain the reason that certain waiting-lists remain so stubbornly high. If elective admissions per 1000 are rising year on year yet waiting-lists remain relatively stable, then (1) people are getting sicker and/or (2) doctors have lowered the threshold for referral and treatment. The same applies to emergency cases. Using these types of indicators there is just a chance that a sensible debate can follow on the cause of waiting-lists etc. Note that a health authority will have to include activity from fundholding practices within its boundaries as increasing amounts of clinical activity move from health authorities' contracts to fundholders with each year. This proviso applies to most reports discussed in this chapter.

Average length of stay

This is a measure already widely used on both sides of the Atlantic.

Average day case cost and day cases per 1000

In a UK setting this should be supplemented with a separate report for outpatients. The formula is similar to the inpatient one previously demonstrated. For example:

Assume: Total day cases in year to date = 6000
Resident population = 220 000
Days in year to date (YTD) = 150
Step 1: Gross days YTD = 6000 ÷ (150 ÷ 365)
= 6000 ÷ 0.410
= 14 634
Step 2: Day cases/1000 in YTD = 14 634 ÷ (220 000 ÷ 1000)
= 14 634 ÷ 220
= 66.53

Therefore day cases/1000 residents for the YTD = 66.53.

The above, in combination with the inpatient reports are recommended for inclusion in the standard reporting set for health authorities. For the more ambitious, case mix-based variants of the above reports would be extremely useful. These would help to answer some of the questions that arise when actual activity and costs show a variation from budget, e.g.: 'Our cost per case is rising, is that a result of a heavier than expected case mix?'

It is recommended that these become nationally reported data sets, thus tackling a chronic problem for those seeking to compare performance and clinical practice in the NHS – lack of consistency in definitions and reporting (an indefensible weakness for a state-run national health care system). Readers considering the use of the above indicators are advised to bear in mind the following:

- decide what definitions you want to use before starting data collection and analysis

- try to get neighbouring authorities to undertake the same work and agree to share the results – a lack of benchmarks is frustrating and limits the value of the information

- remember to include activity and costs howsoever purchased. This includes private hospital activity and extracontractual referrals both of which may not be recorded in the normal manner in central returns.

Health authorities have an opportunity and responsibility to develop a role for themselves in the provision of timely and accurate information on actual and comparative performance using GPs/GP practices as the building-blocks of their reporting. The challenges in establishing a reporting mechanism which can produce, disseminate and then respond to such information on a regular (probably monthly) basis are considerable. Even HMOs, with their considerable investment (by UK standards) in staffing and IT, find it difficult to meet the demands for such information. They also agonize over whether to anomize practices in reports, whether league tables are catalysts for change or are counterproductive, whether to turn around reports quickly (but risk errors) or wait another month for a more complete (but less timely) picture. There is no 'correct' answer to these questions, but it is clear that information drives the practice of medicine.

Purchasers (on both sides of the Atlantic) need to ask themselves if they have a sufficient infrastructure to meet likely demand in this area. This level of provision needs to become routine before the service turns its attention to the 'holy grail' of health service informatics – the development and analysis of longitudinal health records for individuals and population groups.

Whilst it remains a legitimate criticism of nearly all health care information (on both sides of the Atlantic) that they provide only snapshots of health status and disease systems through concentrating on discrete (largely acute) episodes of care, the barriers to producing such information in a systematic and replicable manner are formidable. The problems in the USA were touched upon in the previous chapter when discussing the difficulties in producing outcome data. However, much as we rail against the frustrations of our current systems, we must realize that we have some way to go in exploiting their current potential. We would serve patients, public and ourselves better if we learnt to utilize our existing systems fully before embarking on more ambitious and less certain areas of IT expenditure. Too many meetings with clinicians to discuss important issues (such as patterns of referral and the rising levels of emergency admissions) are based on conjecture, not facts. HMOs and health authorities can act as facilitators on these issues if they have the wherewithal to fill this gap.

Likewise, debate on contracts will remain firmly rooted in the realm of prices and volume until the providers are prepared to release information which allows judgements to be made on clinical processes and their outcomes. These have to be sufficiently comparable with other providers' reporting to allow 'the consumer' to arrive at a sensible verdict on cost vs quality issues. It has already been noted that US health care institutions have a paucity of real data on patient outcomes and costs (as most accounting systems report revenues against charges – not costs). They are being forced down this road through a mixture of competitive pressure from other providers, and the attentions of purchasers (HMOs, Medicare, etc.), including employer groups.[53] When one considers that back in 1989 Chrysler Corporation estimated that health care costs added $700 to the cost of each vehicle compared to $246 in Japan and $223 in Canada, the surprise is that pressure for more progress in this area is not greater.[54]

In the NHS the cost/volume/quality matrix is given added focus by the role government plays in allocating resources and setting targets. Without better information concerning the relationship of one factor to another, there is likely to be a continued drive for greater volume and lower prices. As the next chapter helps to illustrate, where the system of performance management is such that executives can be asked to do almost anything in the name of a central policy directive, the lack of robust information for measuring the impact on the service being offered to patients has to be worrying.

7

The business process

Old actions speak louder than new words

Anon.

This chapter compares certain elements of the conduct of business in the NHS and in US health care. In many respects it has been the most difficult part of the book to write. Much of it is necessarily subjective and almost anecdotal in nature. An individual's exposure to different systems of management is necessarily limited – in the author's case to an NHS career for the most part spent in Wales (which has a distinctive organizational structure) and experience in the USA drawn from only one company. Certain differences in management style and culture are subtle and the danger is that in attempting to draw these out, one slips into characterization and generalities. However, this is too important an area to pass over as reform of the management process, perhaps more than any other single element described in this book, will determine the ability of the NHS (outside funding issues) to deliver quality services to the nation. Much of what has been observed is thought to be generally applicable.

Certain observations and conclusions may be considered deliberately provocative – particularly the section on the relationship between health authorities, civil servants and their political masters. Some may consider this an exercise in polemic; yet the director of the Health Division, Welsh Office (the senior civil servant accountable for NHS Wales) recently acknowledged that all parties need to 'adjust to the new world' and that 'the emphasis must change to a dialogue about aims and related results and what the department can do to help Authorities achieve them'.[55] As examined below, the impact of the civil service culture and the command and control mindset it typically generates go a long way towards explaining the differences in health care management between the two countries. It remains to be seen if all parties can successfully 'adjust to the new world'.

The author was hoping (unrealistically) that a study of management techniques in the USA would reveal a 'brave new world' of textbook efficiency and informed decision-making. After all, Sentara is a highly successful company operating in a commercial environment with a considerable reputation Stateside for innovation and entrepreneurial behaviour. Unfortunately there were no miracle cures. Indeed, the company's management team share some of the same concerns one hears every day within the NHS – too many meetings, poor preparation, overloaded agendas, too many conflicting priorities, inadequate information, too great an emphasis on short-term results etc. Direct observation supported those concerns and perhaps the NHS can draw comfort from this – although not from the fact that Sentara was tackling these issues and the underlying business processes via considerable investment in company-wide reengineering (see Appendix V) and restructuring at a time when the cost of NHS reorganization is having to be met from existing resources.

The fact that such radical measures are having to take place at all, across a whole range of industries, shows that the commercial sector is not years ahead of the NHS in these matters. Improvements are possible and should be enacted, but this is not a case of the bureaucratic tortoise and the commercial hare – except inasmuch as the NHS has the theoretical capacity to catch up (if not overtake) commercial industry, because its managerial infrastructure is generally leaner. Consider the figures below.

Commissioning authorities are currently set a 1% operating cost against total revenues, with further savings expected each year through 'efficiencies'. Sentara's Managed Care Division alone had almost $36 million budgeted for 'administration' costs in the financial year 1995/6, which represented a 22.39% increase on the previous year. Overall its administrative costs were around 15% of the premium dollars it received – its income. In contrast commissioning authorities (and trusts) should be better able to achieve best practice in terms of the conduct of meetings etc., simply because their organizations are so much more streamlined. Nevertheless, current practice remains considerably removed from 'best practice' and one may be forced to conclude that 'best practice' will remain elusive given the public sector/civil servant mindsets and conventions in which the NHS currently operates.

Sentara Health System was atypical of many US health care companies in that it was an integrated system – it owned hospitals and nursing homes, operated community services and primary care centres, and had a managed care operation. In UK terms, it had a number of purchaser and provider functions within one company. This appeared to give it greater organizational overheads than is the norm for US industry. There was periodic questioning amongst Sentara's management of the wisdom of maintaining such a structure, with the organizational problems it created often being cited. There remains a tension between the advantages integration can give for leverage across the entire system vs the greater focus, autonomy and streamlining that are thought to exist through splitting such a company up. This mirrors somewhat the debate between internal market enthusiasts and traditionalists in the UK.

Meetings

In the USA, meetings are characterized by being generally to the point with good time discipline. They are not used for interdepartmental bickering and point-scoring. There is very strong team emphasis. There is little waffle – they are usually focused on specific issues – and there is a notable absence of any deliberate withholding or misrepresentation of financial or other information.

On the down side, there are too many meetings, often overlapping and often involving the same core people (possibly a symptom of inadequate delegation and a desire to obtain consensus). There is a tendency to use meetings to convey information whilst at the same time moving through agendas at a rate that does not allow complex issues to be fully considered and decisions taken. This sometimes leads to decisions being revisited. Agendas and papers are often tabled rather than circulated in advance, and notes of the meeting are by no means always produced.

Senior managers also devote a lot of time to meetings/events outside the company – congressman-briefing breakfasts, alliances with other companies, business community events etc. Overall all levels of management think there are too many meetings, and too much time spent at them. This leads to a kind of collective guilt about spending any time discussing issues, which in turn can lead to a requirement to hold further meetings! In the opinion of the author, this is aggravated by a tendency to avoid exchanges in meetings that might threaten 'team spirit'.

In the NHS, there is a stronger tradition of prepared agendas and pre-circulated notes/papers, and more time is taken to explore issues. On the other hand, there are also too many meetings, often overlapping, with poor time management. Unless chairmanship is particularly strong there is a tendency towards 'civil war' and revisiting issues. Financial information is often weak. There is an inadequate sense of corporate responsibility to understand information being presented outside the sphere of one's own profession – in stark contrast to the situation in the USA. There remains the suspicion that the dynamics of certain groups in the NHS are such that meetings are used as a means of avoiding decisions.

In both systems key personnel have an extended number of 'external' meetings to attend which are largely unavoidable. Key staff typically put in long hours and have reached the point of diminishing returns in attempting to do more by working harder. Ways have to be found to work 'smarter'. In this context it means following time management and organizational rules which are widely known but seldom fully implemented:

- ensure objectives of any meeting are well defined and the chair is clear what is to be achieved. Keep succinct notes with responsibilities clearly defined

- only hold a meeting if there is no practical alternative. Make everyone clear about the costs of meeting

- using meetings to convey information should be the exception, not the rule. Be very aggressive about using e-mail and/or notice boards to inform

- other than in exceptional circumstances precirculate papers and agendas

- weed out 'passengers' – limit participants but not participation

- delegate

- important issues deserve a decent discussion. Make time for such items, perhaps via regularly scheduled 2–3 hour 'retreats'. These should not be talking shops – decisions should be made

- eliminate non-essential activity: results come from doing the right thing, not doing things right

- do not accept substandard performance – if the organization accepts mediocrity it will get just that

- there should only be one quarterback on the field and the team rallies to the calls he or she makes! This should set the tone both for meetings and the general conduct of business.

Management philosophy

In the words of one US executive:

> Mistakes are part of the currency of decision-making. We pay people to make decisions and usually they're good ones. As long as the bad ones aren't terminal and the lessons are learned, we move on because if you play too safe in this business – take no risks and don't test the envelope – you're going to be left behind. Being left behind *is* unacceptable.

Contrast this with the advice I was given by a senior manager on my first day as a trainee in the NHS: 'Never make a decision today which you can put off 'till tomorrow'.

All US health care companies have one thing in common – they emphasize the importance of a strong management team. The management process, Wall Street and the discipline of the market demand this to be the case. The emphasis is firmly on leadership. Because of this there is no real tradition of US management acting in a subservient way to clinicians – although this should not be confused with the considerable professional independence doctors have historically enjoyed whilst health care in the USA experienced decades of continuous growth and profits.

Many US companies are working hard to integrate clinicians into their decision-making process, but this should not be confused with any dilution of managerial accountability or responsibility. Culturally, US management is highly entrepreneurial in temperament, with a genuine belief in its ability to determine the company's (and their own) future.

This makes for a refreshing change from the traditional NHS mindset which has risk-avoidance at its core. Frustration at the service's inability to chart its own destiny is compounded by an unfortunate characteristic – first observed by Enoch Powell (Minister of Health 1960–3) – of being best able to obtain additional resources not through success, but by an ability to draw attention to how awful things are:[56]

> One of the most striking features of the National Health Service is the continual, deafening chorus of complaint which rises day and night from every part of it, a chorus only interrupted when someone suggests that a different system altogether might be preferable, which would involve the money coming from some less (literally) palpable source. The universal Exchequer financing of the service endows everyone providing as well as using it with a vested interest in denigrating it, so that it presents what must be a unique spectacle of an undertaking that is run down by everyone engaged in it.

Another characteristic of NHS general management has been its inability to define a belief and value system outside that handed down to it by government. In this it betrays its administrative historical roots – a role which emphasized passive guardianship of others' decisions. As a result, it is difficult to avoid the conclusion that neither the NHS nor its managers have a 'management philosophy' as such.

Organizational structure

One might be forgiven for thinking that the management structures and organizational principles of the commercial sector would be a significant reference point for those who set in train the general reorganization of the

NHS – and of late the purchasing function. There are valuable lessons from the commercial world for an NHS which has always struggled to inject any real leadership and dynamism into the management process, but unfortunately these have been for the most part simply ignored.

The central problem is the propensity of politicians, aided by civil servants, to dictate structures and process, instead of setting out key objectives (ends) and leaving the means to the people who know best – those engaged in operations. Politicians have no practical experience in this matter – although they are not short of opinions – and senior civil servants approach the issue with a mindset generally at odds with the kind of creative solutions required for a fast-changing industry. This type of control and command mentality might best be described as anally retentive governance.

The NHS is exhorted to be businesslike. Each constituent part of the NHS – the executive, health authorities and trusts – tell the public (and themselves) that they aspire to be businesslike. The author believes these aspirations are unlikely to be fulfilled in what remains at heart a control-and-command management system.

When I returned from six months in the USA, in January 1996, I was struck (but also unsurprised) both at how little had been done to prepare authorities for the April reorganization and by the fact that the general morale of the workforce in Wales seemed lower than when I had left it. Low investment, poor morale and planning blight are not characteristics shown by many 'businesslike' organizations (or at least those intending to remain in business very long). Those charged with taking the reorganization forward (a very difficult task for any organization) were shouldered with unnecessary additional burdens. Commercial companies are not immune from poorly executed reorganizations (although I know of none which would attempt such major changes without setting aside sums to assist restructuring) but their penalty is likely to be competitive disaster. The NHS does not face the same disciplines – and it shows.

'Know who your customer is': the motto of business is the key to understanding the NHS 'business' process and why it is unlikely to emulate the private sector. Chief executives, non-executives and line managers know who their ultimate customer is: the government. Whilst this view remains, the NHS will not operate in a truly 'businesslike' fashion because governments (of almost any political persuasion) value conformity, are risk-adverse and normally operate within an ideological framework. Most businesses value profits, which they consider best secured through customer satisfaction; they are risk-takers and ideological pragmatists. Sometimes the public and the government share the same values and priorities. On these occasions NHS organizations, operating to political directives, appear to be 'businesslike', 'responding to the market' and 'customer-focused'. When the priorities diverge these same organizations are castigated as public-sector dinosaurs. In truth they respond on each occasion to the same drum. The beat may change, but the drummer remains the same. By commercial standards the NHS remains customer-oriented (with the exception of the 'customer' referred to above) in the same way sausage factories are pig-oriented. In part this is a natural consequence of running a health service which is operating at an artificially low level of income in relation to demand. US health care quality orientation (as measured by the public if not by health economists) reflects its capacity to 'grow the cake'. The impact of this on the business process in each country is considerable.

Management development

Belasco and Stayer advise us to 'focus on the skills required to do the job that needs to be done. Background is secondary and relevant only as it supports performance in this job.'[57]

Unlike in the USA, there is a growing concern over the ability of the service (and particularly health authorities) to grow the next generation of senior executives. For example, the advertisement for the only non-professional executive director positions (director of contractor services) in the 1996 Welsh reorganization emphasized not general management skills but the particular body of knowledge normally associated with a narrow set of traditional FHSA duties:

> With a thorough knowledge of primary care and matters relating to the statutory responsibility for administering and monitoring the independent contractor professions, you will take a leading role in ensuring that primary healthcare issues are appropriately recognised in all aspects of the Authority's work.

The accumulated effects of the uncertainty that has been visited upon the NHS commissioning function are such as to deter many of the most promising managers and trainees from making a career within these organizations. Hospitals are viewed as a safer bet ('they won't be able to legislate them out of existence') and a faster, more certain career track. This is exactly the opposite of what is happening in the USA where the best students and the most ambitious managers are joining managed care companies.

In both countries it is the 'purchasing' function – broadly defined – that is pushing back the envelope and engendering change. The function requires the brightest and the best. In the USA it attracts such people. In the UK this is undermined by (barely camouflaged) hostility to 'management'.

This transcends party barriers, not least because no one ever lost votes tilting at bureaucratic windmills. The NHS is expected to emulate the best practices of industry but there is neither the recognition, nor the nurturing of the necessary culture and infrastructure to achieve the desired results.

The author is not saying that the reorganization of the NHS purchasing should not have occurred. The principal aim – to create a wholly new organization from the health authorities and FHSAs – is both sensible and long overdue. We may have organizations with some real potential to leverage change. They have size and hence some critical mass on their side. They are no longer hamstrung by artificial boundaries (forgetting the social services issue for the moment) and because there are fewer of them they can more easily enter into productive alliances.

Notwithstanding the above, the basic organizational building-blocks of the NHS – GP practice, NHS trusts, health authorities – are very small by US standards. The trend in the US is clearly towards that of buy-outs and amalgamations. Health care companies are getting bigger and bigger. Some 'purchaser' organizations are truly huge affairs with millions of 'covered lives' throughout the USA. Multihospital chains are also common with 'independents' (similar in size to the smaller NHS trusts) isolated, commercially under threat and reducing in numbers. As previously noted, even doctors tend to be organized in multipractice partnerships, with many in turn being members of an IPA comprising hundreds or even thousands of doctors.

Sentara, with a turnover approaching $1 billion and over 10 000 staff, four acute hospitals, etc., was no more than a medium-sized health care company by US standards. One of its principal concerns was to grow sufficiently (either directly or via strategic alliances) to allow it to fight off potential competition from larger companies. The conventional wisdom of the US executives would be that NHS organizations (in all areas) are too small and fragmented to operate effectively in such a complex environment as health care. They lack critical mass, whether that is measured clinically, managerially or financially.

Sutton's law

What areas do US health care executives concentrate their energies in? Essentially, there is a simple answer. They follow the bankrobber Willy Sutton's advice and 'go where the money is'. The organizational structure of the companies, their information systems and use of time reflect this. As part of this same philosophy there is a considerable investment in IT and information staffing. Its companies know that modern health care is information-intensive. Good decisions need to be both timely and informed. Investment in IT and information services is based on these sound business principles.

Sentara's policy on management development is also of interest. Whilst it was prepared to recruit externally where it was felt necessary, it also tried to retain and develop its staff. It tried to recruit staff with a view to them having a long-term career with Sentara (whilst being prepared to transfer them from division to division within the company). The question has to be posed how such a long-term view is going to be retained in an NHS where executive life-expectancy is perceived to be short and largely dependent on the achievement of short-term goals. The author was recently informed that the average tenure of a trust chief executive in England was less than two years. One hopes this is incorrect, but the question is whether organizations are generally behaving as if this were the case. Why invest in staff (beyond altruism and vision) if you consider yourself unlikely to be a beneficiary of the long-term development of your organization?

The corporate role

In the words of one US executive: 'The future is OK. It's the transition that will kill you'.

There is no equivalent of the health authority/region/civil service relationship at Sentara. The company has a corporate headquarters and certain 'corporate' functions; but there is a fundamental difference in the way the civil service mediates its relationship with the NHS and the role of a corporate entity in a company like Sentara. Essentially the American touch is lighter, in that there is considerably greater autonomy, and priorities are more clearly articulated (although criticism can be levelled about relative performance in this area, principally due to the inherent tendency to dilute attention across divisions when operating as an integrated system). However, a significant comment was heard at a meeting (attended by the vice presidents representing each division of the company) when the president/chief executive officer talked about the need to meet the targets set for financial performance. He said: 'We can get back on course': and it is significant that he said 'we', not 'you'. One might summarize relationships between the centre and its agents in the UK with a similarly pithy expression: 'We'll tell you when you're doing it wrong'.

This, and the relative absence of press and public scrutiny were two of the most profound differences encountered whilst working in the USA. Neither typically gets the attention they deserve – perhaps being seen as necessary evils. Of the former it is difficult to see how authorities can be expected to conduct their affairs in a manner akin to best practice until this relationship is reformed. Historically these relationships have been poor and unless they are improved the NHS can never be 'all that it can be'.

This is an uncomfortable subject – especially for a system which still sets considerable store on 'the chain of command' – but leaving the relationship unexamined would mean overlooking one of the key factors in explaining why NHS management can appear dysfunctional in comparison with the private sector.

Whilst it may be unreasonable to expect health authorities and trusts to operate at the cutting edge of business practice, there should be a justified expectation that any review process between these entities and the 'centre' will follow established commercial practice. As a participant in accountability reviews, the author regrets to say that no better example could be given of the need to reform the relationship between these bodies. The accountability review is billed as the primary process by which an authority's progress against objectives is assessed. It is meant to be essentially a retrospective look at the year just gone but unsurprisingly time is also spent talking about current and future objectives. This is reasonable. What is less so is the expectation that this can be achieved in a couple of hours when so much time will be devoted to ritualistic presentations and questions from various professional/interest groups and where so little time is spent discussing financial and service reconfiguration issues. As a result, the accountability review process highlights the pressing need for reform of the business (sic) process between the centre and its agents.

The presence of the CHCs (health 'watchdogs' which, in part, are meant to represent the views of local people) illustrates the confusion over what the review should be for. If the views of local CHCs on an authority's performance are required (which is an entirely legitimate concern), then they should meet the executive separately from the authority. Accountability reviews should not be exercises in public relations, but like most multi-agency meetings they carry the seeds of self-deception through the people invited to participate and the items for discussion. This is not the 'American way', nor is it businesslike. Any meaningful reform of the management process must start here ... physician heal thyself.

Strategic planning

According to Alan Kennedy, writing about the Italian army under Mussolini, 'its collective inefficiency, lack of initiative, and concern for personal career prospects was stultifying ... Dominated by its cautious and inadequately trained senior officers ... [its leader] was a strategical liability of the first order'.[58] No doubt some readers would have thought Kennedy was writing about the NHS. Is this judgement too harsh when it comes to the planning process?

Strategic planning appears to have temporarily gone out of fashion in the NHS. The current emphasis is on altogether snappier, focused texts, and to the degree that there already existed forests of bloated verbiage as unread as it is unimplementable, this is no bad thing.

What is yet to replace the old strategic plan and its accompanying processes is a document that relates to one's particular business environment and sets challenging but realistic objectives. A plan that is going to be of use to an organization acknowledges at the outset the need to prioritize and with it the necessity of trade-offs between desirable but conflicting objectives. Historically, strategy formulation in the NHS at both national and local level has a particularly poor record in this regard. A commercial enterprise that served up as many conflicting messages and priorities as the NHS has at present would be in serious trouble. It invites paralysis through overload. As children we are taught that we cannot have everything. We have to learn to be patient and live with our choices. If a strategy does not have this at its core it is likely to be worse than useless.

The strengths of the planning process in the commercial world (as seen in Sentara) lay in their ability to act on the above principles. The number of company failures in any year should serve as a reminder that many commercial plans are far from being uniform examples of 'best practice'. Many commercial plans (both good and bad) are distinguished by a conscious desire for flexibility. This can be a double-edged sword. On the one hand, strategy should not become a millstone in a fast-changing environment. On the other, a call for flexibility can act as a less than subtle device for U-turns at the first sign of a setback. As a side note, actually finding strategic documents at Sentara was not easy as there was a reluctance to commit to paper commercially sensitive information. This made formulation and communication of strategic goals heavily reliant on a verbal process (somewhat to the consternation of the author)!

The general lesson for the NHS is the need to strike a balance (never easy) between short-term performance issues and longer-term goals. Prior to about 1990, there was inadequate attention given to performance issues, which also impacted on the ability of the service to take forward its strategic objectives. Of late the pendulum has swung the other way with short-term considerations very much in the ascendency: hence the current obsession with the Patient's Charter performance and league tables. As a result, insufficient attention is given to the longer-term consequences of an 'activity driven' health service.

The advent of GPs as major players in both strategy formulation and implementation does not make this process any easier. Nor will it eliminate the need for strategic planning and decisions. How these will come about is less than clear – although there is clearly an expectation that health authorities will be accountable for coordinating this process and delivering coherent policies.

Although there can be no miracle cures – regardless of organizational structure – the task is likely to be made easier if all parties (civil service, authorities, trusts and GPs) believe they are 'singing from the same hymn sheet'. It has to be *our* strategic plan and *our* success.

Capital planning

Compared with the USA the NHS suffers from acute under-capitalization. Overall its capital stock is declining as evidenced by the backlog of statutory maintenance and equipment in need of replacement. Moreover, there is evidence that some of the modest increase in revenue funding made available to the NHS has come via transfers from the capital monies. It was recently reported that the NHS capital budget is to be cut by nearly £400 million (the current allocation is about £2 billion) in the next three years.[59] The expectation is that the private sector will plug most of the gap. Yet neither the creation of the internal market nor the recently announced 'private finance initiative' (PFI) has made, or is likely to make, any fundamental difference to the chronic funding difficulties of the service. The PFI may bring greater discipline into the capital planning process, but the small number of projects attractive enough to draw private financing mean that it is likely to prove difficult to obtain capital from traditional sources (given the capital to revenue transfers). The scale of the problem starts to become apparent when one considers that for 1997/8 alone the government is relying on the private sector to contribute £170 million compared with £47 million for 1996/7. This is an increase in private money of 242% in real terms. Meanwhile, for the previous ten years total backlog maintenance in the NHS has remained unaltered at about £2.4 billion.[60]

There is a truly puzzling paradox concerning many capital projects in the NHS. Despite the general level of under-capitalization there remain capital monies for approved schemes for which there is an insufficient case for development and an inadequate revenue source to support them. How does this occur and would total fundholding/GP commissioning prevent such schemes from occurring? They occur primarily due to the interplay of three factors.

First, as previously stated, capital is a relatively scarce commodity and organizations have to compete with each other for what is available. However, in a system where all capital submissions for a defined part of the country are being assessed by one body, there is an inevitable tendency to allocate monies over time in a way that ensures 'everyone gets their turn'. This is defendable – not least from an equity standpoint – but also means that when an organization thinks its 'turn' is coming up there is an understandable desire to put forward a scheme (typically one that costs a lot of money). This often means dusting off plans for a capital development that have existed for some time – a new hospital or ward block, for example – which forms part of an 'approved' strategy regardless of its current relevance (this is where agreeing to unrealistic but agreeably worded strategies can come back to bite you).

Second, many trusts are still in an expansionist mode of thinking. As new organizations they may believe their future prosperity depends on growth, often at the expense of neighbouring hospitals. Capital schemes bring prestige (and, it is to be hoped, revenues too) to the organization. They are popular with both the staff and public. Moreover, they have been typically part of a strategic plan for some time and have taken on the characteristics of 'a promise'.

Third, to those charged with administering it, the capital planning process is somewhat akin to a sausage machine. Each year monies are allocated as capital resources and the view taken that a good job is one that ensures it is spent within the prescribed timescales and in the prescribed manner. It is less than clear whose job it is to ensure that it is spent wisely. The process essentially becomes one of ticking the right boxes. Once started, there is pressure on all parties to play their part. In the case of the commissioners, this essentially means supporting the scheme in question. The requirement for purchaser support is rightly emphasized in the capital approval process. If authorities are doing their jobs properly, they should review each scheme and, where necessary, state they oppose a scheme. Why does this not happen more often? The failure to conduct a thorough review and state unequivocally one's concerns are rationalized in the following ways (with varying degrees of justification):

- it is in the strategy and we cannot say it is not now relevant without looking foolish

- it will create a public outcry

- the minister/politicians support the scheme

- it is going to be approved anyway

- it is only a paper exercise

- it is at the trusts' own risk, they know our financial situation

- we have no time to review the proposal

- the GPs support it

- who knows if it will increase costs, nobody understands capital charges

- we will approve it because we probably will not be here by the time the thing comes on line.

At its core is the problem that the NHS still operates in a mindset of capital being a 'free good'. The PFI initiative frustrates the NHS because it has built-in further delays – and with it a kind of guaranteed obsolescence for capital projects. Overall, however, as Black notes: 'There is no evidence that the obsession with investing in bricks, mortar and equipment is waning – nor is there evidence that these investments are improving the population's health.'[60]

The other question was whether the devolution of purchasing to GPs would change or improve anything? The most likely answer is that, if anything, it will make matters worse. First, approval from each practice (in their role as purchasers) will in theory be required. This will increase the time pressures on all parties. Second, as previously noted, many GPs give a high priority to protecting and enhancing local services. They will be tempted to view all such capital developments in a favourable light unless the financial and service implications are made very clear to them, and they share the burden of resolving such issues.

If, however, capital projects in the future arise from a sustained dialogue between purchaser(s) and provider in which GPs take the time to take a lead role, the process will be much improved. The problem at root is solvable not by GP involvement in general, or fundholding in particular, but by a much needed injection of realism and financial discipline.

Economies of scale

The primary organizational trend in US health care is the creation of larger managed care/insurance companies through amalgamation or buyouts. The driving force for this is the view that when it comes to negotiating with providers 'God is on the side of the big battalions'. The theory goes that only large companies have the highly desirable characteristics of high member volume, deep pockets (in a business with significant barriers to entry and a requirement for considerable reserves), and management and systems strength in depth. Central to this proposition, however, is the axiom that there is little point in being big (with its attendant disadvantages) if you are not going to make use of the economies of scale and resources commensurate with your size. We shall call this an ability to leverage the gains of being a corporate entity.

A singular inability to obtain such leverage has been an enduring characteristic of the NHS. In key respects the UK's health service does not act as a national entity at all. Rather it resembles, through its patchwork of health authorities (and now trusts), a series of fiefdoms. The most accurate (and colourful) analogy available is that it resembles the Holy Roman Empire which was notable for being neither Holy, Roman, nor an Empire!

This particular organizational form is also notable for what is considered a suitable subject for central direction and what can safely be left in local hands. This can best be illustrated by noting that at one point health authorities in Wales had to get the personal approval of the secretary of state for Wales to replace even a part-time typist, but could effectively develop their own contract currencies. Similarly, on the major issue of health care rationing Virginia Bottomley's (secretary of state for health, 1991–5) stated view was that 'this is a matter for local decision makers'.[61,62]

In summary, the NHS suffers from an inability to obtain sufficient leverage of its corporate resources. The result is that it ends up trying to run a $41 billion enterprise with the organizational methods of two distinct, contradictory and (in this context) equally ineffective mindsets – neurotic micromanagement and the public sector equivalent of the three wise monkeys.

Is current practice relevant?

The NHS business practices reviewed in this chapter have not stood up well to examination. Commercial practices were expected to perform better and largely did, although they are not without their weak areas. How relevant is the NHS analysis if the system is evolving to either a fundholder or GP commissioning-driven system? Most of it remains critical on the basis that:

- the transitional stage is set to last three to five years minimum and in any case a change of government would mean a reevaluation of the fundholding scheme

- the weaknesses highlighted are not particular to health authorities but are systemic. Many of the problems cited are not so much organizational in nature as part of the 'conventional wisdom' of public-sector governance

- the catalyst for the NHS review announced in January 1988, which subsequently led to the creation both of the internal market and fundholding, were well publicized public and professional concerns over funding. Significantly, the review remained silent on this very issue.

Both fundholding and GP commissioning have a number of implicit strengths, but the true test of their organizational structures as a means of taking tough decisions is yet to be tested. It is at that point that any fault lines in the management process will be truly exposed.

Some simple lessons

It is a prerequisite of a successful organization that it has good people working for it and strong leaders who can motivate those around them. Those leaders must have integrity. In the NHS integrity has to transcend mere adherence to established business practice – integrity has to be worn on one's sleeve. However, integrity does not guarantee success. The organization must be able to prioritize its objectives and it has to be prepared to put its best people into areas where there are the biggest problems. For the NHS this translates into an ability to find the best clinicians working in the areas of the greatest deprivation, and the most capable managers working to turn around those places with the biggest problems. With some honourable exceptions this is not the case.

This book has been critical both about the leadership of the NHS and its integrity. There is an absolute requirement for good leaders and the introduction of the Griffiths Report in the early 1980s was a major step forward.[63] Leadership is important. People are an organization's greatest asset. If you fail to look after people the good ones tend to go, leaving a preponderance of dead wood and driftwood. None of this can remotely be classified as rocket science. However, organizations seem to have a hard job learning and – more importantly – acting upon these basic principles.

Finally, there are some issues where leadership is not going to be enough. Leadership alone will not fix the problem. Resources (money) are required and difficult decisions on highly charged issues have to be made. Using half-measures to tackle problems that go to the very core of the enterprise and are integral to its success will not solve the issues, but it will lead to poor morale and a high attrition rate. In this context reorganizations are a symptom of, not solutions to, a wider malaise. *Plus ça change?*

8

Strategic issues in cost-containment

Sometime before 2020 it is likely that we will have the know-how – either already in the clinic or on the way there – to predict, diagnose, and prevent or treat most diseases in most patients

Stuart Davidson MD

We are all strong enough to bear the misfortunes of others

La Rochefoucould

This book has been written to give an insight into particular features of the UK's and USA's system of health care, with a view to supplementing the tools already available to those concerned with shaping and managing health services. This is far from being exclusively the province of professional managers. Implicit throughout the book has been the view that an overreliance on 'political' decision-making and 'cooperative behaviour' to achieve desired outcomes in health care amounts to little more than the unfettered use of political processes to determine matters which can be better settled by a mixture of market forces and clinical logic.

Cooperative restraint as a means of ensuring the status quo is inherently political in nature and, as such, is destined to be internally unsustainable. When politicians call for an end to selfish market-motivated behaviour and instead promote cooperative enterprise (as appears to be the case with Labour) they assume either that markets and market signals are irrelevant, and/or that there are more efficient systems for determining the distribution and management of health care resources. This typically translates into some form of central planning model. Labour has yet to show that its policies amount to more than this and how it will combat what many consider to be the irresistible descent towards crisis and cronism associated with such solutions. Politicians (of all parties) are largely silent about how they would tackle the issues set out in this chapter, and this in a way is not surprising, as they are formidable.

The author is a proponent for using market mechanisms (albeit selectively) and of using a greater range of managerial methods than is currently the norm. However, one can easily overhype both markets and managerialism in health care.

The rest of this chapter takes a step back from the debate concerning the relative merits of managed care, fundholding etc., and asks 'what are the opportunities and limits of cost-containment in modern health care? Here, the primary focus is on the fundamental issue of the limits of health and health care – rather than the merits of a particular delivery system. The complexity and gravity of the issues under consideration only allow them to be sketched out in a book whose principal focus lies elsewhere. Why bother then to discuss these issues at all? There are three possible reasons.

First, the issues are important in themselves. If you are interested in health care or are in the business of delivering health services, reflecting on these issues should be as much part of your intellectual composition as the professional soldier's consideration of questions such as what circumstances make for a just war and what constitutes an acceptable and unacceptable action in pursuit of a valid military objective. It should be apparent that these are not idle philosophical concerns.

Second, neither managed care, fundholding nor any other organizational form operates in a vacuum. This book's broad contention is that managed care and fundholding (or more specifically capitation funding) are the more effective means of constraining health care costs whilst maintaining – and on occasion enhancing – quality. These are not exclusively the only effective means, nor by themselves do they guarantee cost control. Their success and appropriateness are contingent on other, essentially external, factors. Health care systems – their means of funding, delivery and underlying philosophies – are products of their particular society. This helps to explain why you cannot simply transplant the health care system of one country into another.

If the citizens of the USA continue to be prepared to devote considerably in excess of 10% of their gross national product (GNP)* to health care, then managed care, operating in its current environment may well be sufficient to stabilize or even slightly reduce expenditure. However a desire both to provide universal access to health care within an operating budget of say, 8% of GNP or less, would entail more radical changes than just increasing the population covered by managed care. This is not the same thing as saying that managed care is ineffective or that it would have no part to play in a reformed system.

* In 1992 it stood at $838.5 billion or 14% of GNP with the former director of the Office of Management and Budget testifying to Congress that without serious structural changes, health care would account for 17% of GDP by 2000 and 37% by 2030.[54]

Third, from the foregoing it should be apparent that reforming the supply side of health care is important, but to have any realistic expectation of achieving a total solution, attention also has to be given to the demand side of the equation. This chapter therefore concerns itself with ensuring the expectations from health care reform are aligned with reality.

Unless we have realistic expectations of our respective health care systems – what it should cost, what it can and cannot do to combat disease and improve health, what is affordable and who should pay, when death can be cheated and when it is wiser to concede to the inevitable – and can reach some form of consensus, we will lurch from crisis to crisis. Moreover we will be trapped in the unenviable paradox of spending more and more yet being less satisfied with our lot. What then are the key issues?

Overcapacity

This is a significant problem on both sides of the Atlantic. The UK has less of an overcapacity problem than the USA, but can afford it even less, due to its considerably reduced expenditure on services as expressed both absolutely and in relation to percentage of GNP. Given the constant flow of news concerning hot-bedding, patients left on trolleys for hours, closures to admissions due to bed shortages etc., it may seem strange to cite this as a transatlantic issue. Yet overcapacity in the UK (or as often undertaking care in an inappropriate setting) takes two principal forms.

First, there are too many facilities trying to be district general hospitals – that is, hospitals capable of admitting both emergency and elective cases with the support of a full range of clinical specialties (surgery, medicine, orthopaedics, anaesthetics, obstetrics and gynaecology, paediatrics etc. – but not necessarily departments such as nephrology, cardiac surgery or neonatal intensive care). Too often there is insufficient population to support such a specialty mix – despite the significant impact of supplier-induced demand – and these hospitals struggle both in terms of their cost-efficiency and clinical viability.

Typically, these hospitals will also struggle to obtain sufficient income to cover operations because funding to purchasers assumes a more efficient distribution of facilities.

Second, there are too many 'cottage-type' hospitals. Despite their undoubted popularity with local people these are all too often run down buildings with a considerable backlog of statutory and highly desirable maintenance. The suspicion of the private sector that many NHS hospitals would not pass health authority inspection requirements (nursing homes must meet these standards as part of their registration requirements) is by no means unfounded. The typical patient mix in a cottage hospital is often essentially the same as can be found in the average nursing home, plus a splattering of 'respite cases' – which if they should be funded as 'health care' (a highly debatable point) could be done so in a less expensive setting.

The closure of these beds could be readily absorbed by the private sector – which has its own problems with over-supply – with the net result that more elderly patients could be cared for within the same resources. Much of the bed-blocking problem in acute hospitals is due to this type of patient. The UK has yet to align its economic incentives to purchasers, providers and patients sufficiently well to sort this problem out, but the above, whilst not a total solution, will help. Alternatively, the savings from closures and cheaper care, via the private sector, could be invested elsewhere.

This is not occurring more often primarily due to the vocal opposition of local residents, often with support from health staff. For their part, health authorities reflect politicians' nervousness of making such unpopular decisions. Where there is no political will to face up to these issues it effectively becomes impossible to close NHS facilities – as when John Redwood (Secretary of State for Wales 1993–5) made it clear to chief executives that he was personally opposed to closures and endorsed cottage hospitals under the 'small is beautiful' banner. Unfortunately the general public continue to labour under the misconception that beds equal health care – the more you have, the better health care must be – and politicians of all persuasions tend to act both as mirrors and ciphers for public opinion on this issue.

As Spiers notes:[64]

> ... the local hospital remains a source of local loyalties and affection. It represents an idea rather than an institution. It is a representative sign of the integrity of a community, and a vital element in public consciousness. Its recurrence of ritual is a comforting source of continuity, quietude and consolation in a world increasingly dedicated to change. Hence, in part, the lack of social consent for planned and 'needed' change which health authorities 'know' is necessary. Hence, in part, anxiety about 'commercialization', spending on 'image', and increases in management costs. The affection reserved for local community hospitals, and the commitment to universal cover which they represent in the imagination of the nation, is one source of the evident unpersuasiveness of statistics when produced to justify closures. This is the denial of the intuitively untrue.

Interestingly, it is likely that total fundholding would lead to some rapid movement on the second issue (cottage hospitals) whilst the signs are that it will aggravate the former problem – at least in the short term. As previously noted in the section on fundholding in Chapter 4, many GPs attempt to build up local services on the reasonable grounds that this is likely to benefit their patients. The longer-term clinical and financial wisdom of such initiatives often gets obscured. However on the issue of cottage hospitals, devolution of resources to the GP may well lead to a rapid reappraisement of services which in the old model had the perceived twin virtues of being both convenient and 'free'.

GPs are normally well acquainted with nursing and residential homes. Should the economic benefits to the practice of utilizing the private sector become real it is likely that many GPs would rapidly shift ground. GPs, historically one of the foundation stones of opposition to hospital closures, would act as the catalyst for change. This has an additional benefit in that local doctors are considerably more credible voices for change than either 'management' or government. It may be that such facilities will not close but will change their function. They may be used more effectively to prevent admission to acute hospitals and thus deflecting the seemingly remorseless rise in emergency admissions highlighted in Chapter 3. If this is the case, there will be significant clinical and economic knock-on effects for the general hospitals (as is already starting to occur with the shift of some procedures to primary care settings). Once again this is a development where the NHS is following a trend set in the USA.

Turning to the USA, we have some similar dynamics operating, although overt political considerations typically play a subordinate role. State regulatory bodies actually put pressure on health care companies to rationalize capital stock. For example, when Sentara made an application to allow six overnight beds to be incorporated into its Careplex facility (essentially a day case and outpatient unit in UK terminology), the State wanted the company to agree to a reduction of a hundred beds at one of its General Hospitals (about one-third of its licensed capacity) in compensation.

Chronic overcapacity of both the hospital sector and physician offices is common but there is a considerable reluctance to close facilities. Returning to the above example, the reluctance to agree to the regulators' proposal serves to illustrate the general issues at play. The opposition to rationalization revolves around five main factors.

First, closed beds and offices means lost revenue. Once you agree to a closure you are accepting by default that your potential revenue umbrella has shrunk. Never mind that there is little realistic chance that the beds will be occupied.

Second, it is in the nature of companies with large fixed assets to be unduly optimistic about the future of the market – it hurts too much to get out. Substantial fixed assets create barriers to exit. In a sense these become all the more formidable when there is no debt on the capital stock: 'It's all paid for, so let's keep it open and hope that circumstances change'. This dynamic was explored in an article in the business magazine *Fortune* in March 1992 where the focus of attention was the electrical goods market.[65] It could apply equally well to health care except that to date this industry has managed to perform the near miraculous feat of operating in a market with chronic overcapacity yet maintain (for the most part) healthy margins. The quotation can be better read as a chilling prediction of what could still occur:

> A growing number of companies are trapped in killing fields of their own making. To protect investments that are too big to write off, they are forced to pursue market share at all costs. Worse, the one real tactical goal of a price war – to bump off a competitor – is less achievable these days. The losers don't fold; they're acquired by somebody with deeper pockets or file for chapter 11 and keep operating ... The greater the market share the more intent the owner is on preserving it – and the greater the belief that somebody else will give. The whole system encourages management to be optimistic. The bottom line is that there is usually too much capacity.

Third, closures hurt corporate pride. They strike at a company's self image. Boards worry about how the outside world will perceive the action taken ('Company X had to close John Doe Hospital, they must be in trouble').

Fourth, the physician community rarely welcomes a closure, the public even less so. In the USA this can directly impact on physician steerage to your facilities and membership of your plans. Both hurt revenues.

Finally, if high charges to commercial/individual payers can keep a hospital in profit or at least solvent, why rationalize? This relatively small payer segment is making up a disproportionate amount of hospital revenues. In effect they are the foundation on which the system's reputation for choice and the prosperity of US health care rests. It is also a major reason the system has not gone into the pricing meltdown described in the *Fortune* quotation.

Managed care will continue to put pressure to drive out excess capacity up to, but no further than is conducive with satisfying its members on issues of choice whilst ensuring a profit on premiums. This may not be radical enough. For almost the entire post-war period the health care systems of both the USA and UK have bucked economic trends and remained aloof from the general economic truth that overcapacity rapidly leads to price reductions. Of the issues cited in this chapter, overcapacity (along with salaries and the introduction of new drugs and technologies) represents one of the areas more amenable to change. Failure to take up this challenge will play its part in disappointing those hoping cost reductions will result from health care reform.

Recent news from America is considerably more encouraging in this respect than the UK, where the political process has effectively paralysed the system's attempts to address capacity issues. One in 12 US community hospitals either merged, was acquired, or acquired another hospital in 1995, according to a report by the pressure group Public Citizen.[66] Rationalization is likely to follow.

Salary costs

Modern health care is a labour-intensive industry, and it is likely to remain so. This sets absolute limits on productivity gains and makes cost reduction a complex and sometimes disappointedly marginal process. Health care also remains (on both sides of the Atlantic) a bastion of restrictive practices. The issues essentially fall into two areas: inflated salaries and overstaffing.

Inflated salaries

What is an inflated salary? Is there such a thing if you believe salary levels are reflections of supply and demand? This is not an economics textbook, and it is accepted that any assertion that certain salaries are set 'too high' (including by reference to market value) is inherently controversial. However, the assertion is made that inflated income levels are a problem for the US health care system – particularly for doctors, or more accurately for certain specialties. Should cardiac surgeons be able to make $500 000 a year, or cardiologists $250 000?[67] That is a matter of conjecture. Could you get them to work for less? Yes. All commentators agree that there is a surplus of doctors in most US specialties. Weiner estimates these surpluses based on the current and future organization of the health market as shown in Table 8.1.[68]

The issue of inflated salaries for NHS staff is rarely raised in the UK (except in the case of managers who, if the media were to have their way, would not be in employment, less still drawing significant salaries). The author believes that the salary problem for NHS doctors is that they are being paid at an artificially low level. In return, they receive 'privileges' – e.g. lax work practices and schedules, private practice, which undermine the efficiency of the NHS. This is analysed in detail by Yates and has recently been the subject of attention in the national journals.[69,70] The issue itself goes all the way back to 1946 as part of the 'deal' struck between the then Labour government and the medical profession. It is time to strike a new bargain.

Table 8.1: Number of physicians per 1000. (Cardiothoracic surgery is defined here as any open-heart surgery)

Specialty	Number of physicians/1000			
	Current	Mature market	End-stage market	Surplus %
Neurosurgery	1.4	0.2	N/A	86
Plastic surgery	1.7	0.5	0.3	71–82
Cardiothoracic surgery	1.8	0.9	0.6	50–67
Psychiatry	12.0	5.2	4.1	57–66
Cardiology	4.9	3.1	1.7	37–65
Anaesthesiology	9.2	4.7	3.9	49–58
Ophthalmology	5.6	3.4	3.1	39–45
General surgery	10.8	6.9	6.2	36–43
Neurology	2.7	1.7	1.6	37–41
Orthopaedics	6.5	5.1	4.2	22–35

Too many staff

The NHS claims to employ more people than the Red Army. In Norfolk, Virginia, Sentara is the largest employer in the region after the US Navy and the Shipyards. The USA has the additional problem of having significant administrative costs as a direct consequence of its funding and delivery systems (Chapter 3). Significant administrative rationalizations (significant in this context would mean cuts in excess of 25%) are only likely to occur if the kind of reforms outlined earlier in the book become a reality.

Both countries suffer from restrictive practices which remain remarkably immune to change despite initiatives as diverse as reengineering; total quality management and the establishment of self-governing (sic) trusts. Whilst in many cases the personal salaries of care givers are low, the sheer numbers employed typically make employee costs the most significant factor in health care expenditure.

Will either managed care or fundholding/GP commissioning address these issues? To the degree that both are likely to drive and respond to market issues, and in so doing put pressure on providers to reduce costs, the answer is yes. However, these agents can also have a negative influence through their own salary base, staffing and inefficiencies. The fact that practice-based purchasing, in particular, is essentially a series of 'cottage industries', creates particular problems. Yet, as with so much else in health care, concern has to be expressed at the ability of market forces *on their own* to ensure positive change. Whatever their benefits in terms of patient knowledge and devolution of responsibility, GP based models of purchasing naturally incur disproportionate administrative costs.[14]

Medical practice variation

Another transatlantic issue, the phenomenon of unexplained MPV has been the subject of increasing research and debate in the professional journals.[69] Whilst some MPV is probably both inevitable and desirable, its current extent is generally considered a major cause of both the composition and variation in costs and clinical outcomes. There is less consensus on what constitutes optimum clinical practice – which is hardly surprising as where strong consensus typically exists, observed MPV is usually small.[71] The causes of MPV in all health care systems lie in four principal areas.

Uncertainty

MPV is a natural response to the uncertainties of clinical medicine and the human condition. We are not robots. Medicine is not an entirely deterministic discipline of cause and effect. It is not always known what works and why. There may be multiple paths available and indeterminate outcomes. MPV's prevalence reflects the surprisingly small body of non-contentious evidence-based medicine available. We have to promote evidence-based research in order to give a sound foundation on which to counter MPV.

Culture

Due primarily to the above, many clinicians view MPV as natural and are opposed to clinical regimentation via protocols and guidelines. Clinicians have a tendency to be temperamentally, culturally and professionally resistant to such methods of practising medicine. Whatever the merits of such a standpoint it has traditionally had an inadequate counterbalance in the form of pressure from payers, educators, peers or public.

Differences in the quality of clinicians

A distribution of competence was discussed earlier in this book. Clinicians are human beings. Human beings are not uniformly competent even when preselected to certain tasks. This can result in practice variation.

Training, experience and tradition ('That's the way we do it here')

Medical education and clinical experience are not uniform. In their formative years as medical students and in training posts, doctors will be exposed to a range of influences from both teachers and peers on methods of practice, which will be of variable quality. Practices learnt in training are more likely to remain unquestioned by those clinicians who fail to keep up with current literature and are infrequent attenders at peer review and educational functions.

On balance it would seem likely that managed care companies are better equipped to tackle MPV than fundholders/GP commissioners – some of whom will be prime examples of the phenomenon. It should be evident from what has already been written about managed care that the identification and tackling of MPV constitutes one of the principle features of this type of organization. In theory the same could be said of the new health authorities, but there are at least three areas of doubt concerning their ability to discharge such a role:

- are adequate resources available? At its most basic, who is going to fulfil this role? Are there enough staff resources to do so, and do they have adequate training, skills and authority? Are the supporting information systems in place or due to be implemented?

- what means are available to enforce compliance? What incentives and sanctions will be available? What mechanisms are in place or will be set up?

- is there the will to confront the issue?

Introduction of new drugs and technologies

In certain respects a subset of the MPV debate, the manner in which new drugs and technologies are introduced (and existing ones used) illustrates some points worth particular emphasis.[72,73] As a science-based discipline, technological innovation – in which is included 'next-generation' treatments such as gene therapy, genetic vaccines and robot assisted surgery as well as the more traditional advances in MRI, prosthetics and drugs – borders on the inevitable. Technological Ludditism is not being touted as a solution. Rather, the issue is the need to ensure proper evaluation and justification of new technologies and therapies within an evidence-based

environment. This also implies a central regulatory body capable of enforcing moratoriums on the use of the unproven and the uneconomic.

Essentially the same issues reside within the drug arena (which continues
to provide exciting opportunities to make radical changes to traditional
courses of treatment for many diseases), but to these can be added the
particular issues of current variation in volume and usage of brand name
vs generic/cheaper drugs prescribed by clinicians, and the profits generated
by the drug industry. This powerful lobby also has the potential to make
radical changes to health care delivery systems through its growing ability
to change the economics of therapeutic prevention versus surgical treatment
of diseases. As previously noted, this could imply very different organizational
forms from the ones considered in this book.

The drive to improve quality of life and defeat death

The enthusiasm with which clinicians often embrace new technologies etc.
is partly a function of sound marketing, partly a perceived need of
institutions and individuals to 'have the best, be first, and gain an edge
over the competition' and partly (in fairness the largest part) a drive to
push back 'the envelope' a little bit further. In clinical practice this means
increasing diagnostic certainty, making the course of treatment safer, refin-
ing an operating technique or tool, improving the chances of a satisfactory
outcome, and maybe cheating death for a little longer. These are not idle
pursuits. This is the driving motivation that has transformed hospitals
from what George Orwell called the 'antechamber to the tomb' to the
places where man-made miracles can, and do, occur.[74]

In the very first chapter reference was made to the impact of the dynamic to improve quality of life. Western industrialized societies will continue to promote the refinement of therapeutic interventions and our body
of knowledge will continue to grow, allowing us to do more. We will continue to keep pushing back the 'envelope'. This is hardly an environment
conducive to cost reduction or even containment on either side of the
Atlantic, yet it is at the heart of the health care industry's insatiable
appetite for resources. Any system which subsidizes (or even makes free at
the point of consumption) something as highly valued as life itself can
expect a surfeit of demand over supply. Whatever its moral value, it makes
for poor economics.

The drowned and the saved

This is the opposing dynamic at work in society. Its proponents are always controversial and never popular, asserting that the medical profession has developed a blind-spot – some of its members can no longer distinguish the sick from the dying. The result can be futile and costly interventions.

Clinicians do not act this way out of mere caprice, nor are their actions taking place in professional isolation from society as a whole. Rather, they are both a mirror and a shaper of our views and expectations on the subject of our own health and mortality. Moreover, medicine emphasizes the paramount importance of the individual and as such has an uneasy relationship with utilitarian considerations.

Yet if anything the dilemmas posed by capabilities exceeding available resources will grow more acute. The debate is being fuelled by demographics – a growing elderly population and associated imbalance between the consumers of wealth and the working population. As it is, 75% of total health costs are usually incurred by only 10% of the population and this is already heavily slanted towards the elderly. This is a problem facing all western health care systems and there is no technique described in this text that can make much of an impact on such a fundamental issue.

Partial solutions lie in the promotion of 'living wills' and treatment protocols. Much more controversial is the issue of euthanasia and the medico-legal imperatives of defensive medicine. Clearly these are subjects which are beyond any health care system's ability to resolve by and of itself. They require the widest engagement. This is not just a practical requirement but also a moral one. In the words of William L Kissick, MD: 'Health, as a vast societal enterprise, is too important to be solely the concern of the providers of services.'[75]

In the absence of public debate and consensus, doctors are making decisions on these issues – by default. *The Lancet* recently reported the outcome of a study of 6802 seriously ill patients in the USA which concluded that physicians seem to be age-biased when it comes to writing 'do not resuscitate' (DNR) orders.[76] The study showed that more DNR orders are written for persons older than 75 years than for those younger, regardless of the patient's prognosis or treatment wishes. With most orders being written within three days of the patient's death (suggesting that clinicians wait until patients are near death before making plans with them) and DNR orders not written for nearly half of the patients who wanted resuscitation withheld, or who had a less than 5% chance of surviving beyond two months, the process starts to assume the characteristics of a lottery.

In a publicly funded, cash-limited system such as operates in the UK, the issue of explicit rationing of health care becomes inevitable, despite an understandable reluctance to address the subject. In an article in the *British Medical Journal*, the necessity of undertaking the rationing process was emphasized in a system which wishes to provide a National Health Service because 'the NHS cannot provide complete coverage given existing resources'. There also remain 'widespread local variations in access to, and quality of treatments, ranging from sub-fertility and renal services to hip replacements and community services'.[77]

Despite the evidence that these issues need addressing, and the fact that they are not unique to the UK, the British response remains a less than potent mixture of pragmatic indifference and diffusion of responsibility. As a result, the NHS has no national framework for priority setting (rationing) nor a defined package of core services, and no sign that policy makers have any intention of undertaking such an initiative. Klein describes Britain's pragmatism as 'half-baked'.[78] Health authorities' sporadic and limited attempts to limit access to treatments usually meet with a reception with might be characterized as 'career-threatening' at best! Individual decisions are sniped at. Whilst the critiques might have validity such as the observation by Evans that authorities lack logical consistency in their decisions on infertility (by restricting access to treatment for infertility on the grounds that it is a socially constructed need, whilst seemingly content to fund services such as sterilization) they often avoid the consequences of their own observation.[79] That is, if choices have to be made, it is best to 'identify all the relevant issues, analyse them publicly and comprehensively, and satisfy all interested parties that their views are being considered'.[80] The subtitle of Evans' article was 'Purchasers should avoid the moral high ground'. The alternative to 'moral' considerations is that access should be denied only on the basis of sound evidence that the treatment is harmful, ineffective or uneconomic to provide. However formed, a stand needs to be taken and that will require the courage to find some form of ground and 'hold the line'.

As for the USA, one has to live there for a time to understand fully how at ease the average citizen is with rationing by income, and how outraged most get at any suggestion that government – or more correctly a government agency – should undertake the rationing process (in such a context it should be remembered that the much publicized Oregon rationing initiative was solely concerned with access to health care by Medicaid recipients).[81]

At its most fundamental level, most Americans have no desire for a 'rational' distribution of resources if such an idea implies any process other than the ability to use individual purchasing power to achieve such an objective. Within the health care arena this translates into a profound desire not to operate a system which provides equity of access. Such a notion undermines the basis on which the 'American dream' was founded – the rise of the individual, and the cruel egalitarianism of the dollar. Perhaps this, as much as anything, suggests that the two countries' health care systems whilst moving closer together, will never meet in the middle – or be entirely comfortable with one another's operating principles.

Conclusion

These are some of the fundamental issues in health care, to which could be added questions such as 'who pays?' and 'what are the legitimate responsibilities of the individual in terms of maintaining their own health?' In the face of these issues, concerns over the level of copayments or the precise method for reimbursing doctors have to be seen as important but still essentially secondary issues. This may seem an unusually self-deprecating way to conclude a book that has spent much of its time focusing on such issues, but it may put current health care reform in its proper perspective.

It should also be apparent that there is a pressing need for leadership and vision as opposed to simply administration – or even just management. This exists more in health care than in most other areas of society because of its inherent complexity, the rate of change, the adverse consequences of poor decisions and the benefits to mankind of getting it right.

US hospital contract

Set out below is an example of some of the key features one might expect to find in a 'typical' US contract between a managed care company and a hospital. Such a contract is not reproduced in detail, primarily because it has all the representative features of a legal document: somewhat wordy, unilluminating and tedious to read. Instead, the principal sections are described so as to illustrate its different focus and subject matter in certain areas from its NHS equivalent.

The list below is illustrative and is far from exhaustive:

1 Definitions

As a legal document enforceable through the courts (as opposed to internal NHS 'contracts' which have no legal status outside of the service), a US contract will normally have been drafted or screened by lawyers. It will contain a definitions section of the parties themselves and key contractual terms – 'copayment', 'IPA', etc.

2 Rendition of care

This section describes the hospital's principal responsibilities in the provision of care to the plan's members. Examples of standard text are given below. The language can appear almost vague on occasion. This is unlikely to be accidental, reflecting counsel's advice: for example the use of the clause expecting services 'consistent with a high standard of competence' and 'in conformity with accepted health care practices prevailing from time to time in the community' without setting out what those standards are, as this might create a liability in itself – either because the standards themselves may be challenged or through failure to comply with them. Thus:

> Upon prior authorization by Plan (except in the case of an emergency), Hospital shall provide to each member all of the Hospital services covered

under this Agreement which are ordered by IPA physicians (or another physician to which patient has been referred by an IPA physician) and which it is licensed to provide. In connection with the provision of Hospital services, Hospital shall use its best efforts in rendering quality Hospital Services in order to provide such services in conformity with accepted health care practices prevailing from time to time in the community and in accordance with Hospital Services required to be provided by the Group agreement, and consistent therewith, Hospital shall perform its obligation hereunder in accordance with a high standard of competence, care and concern for the welfare and needs of members, and in a manner that is dignified and personal.

Hospital shall maintain full licensure and comply fully with all applicable federal, state and local laws and regulations. Hospital shall promptly notify Plan of any action taken against it with respect to such licensure or compliance with laws and regulations, including, but not limited to, any revocation, suspension or enforcement action related thereto.

Hospital shall maintain full accreditation by the Joint Commission on Accreditation of Health Care Organizations. Hospital shall promptly notify Plan of any action taken against it with respect to the Hospital's accreditation by the Joint Commission.

Hospital shall cooperate and communicate with other persons caring for members and provide relevant formation and data requested by Plan, another Plan Hospital, an IPA or an IPA physician in a manner consistent with Hospital policy. Information provided will be limited to that which is usually and reasonably available in the normal operation of Hospital.

Hospital shall participate in a quality and utilization review system established by the Plan, the primary purpose of which shall be to evaluate the quality of health services provided to members and to monitor the utilization of such services by members. This system may include preadmission certification and concurrent review.

3 Eligibility

This section makes clear that the Plan will establish specific procedures to enable the hospital to determine whether a person is eligible for coverage and the nature and extent of that coverage. The hospital must follow these (except in an emergency) prior to commencement of treatment. Failure to do so renders the Plan no longer 'liable to Hospital for any services rendered to persons not authorised as provided in Plan's procedures'.

4 Fiscal relationships

Fiscal relationships cover the methods and forms of payment. Unless some form of capitation arrangement is in effect payment would typically only be made upon presentation of a detailed bill. Thus:

> As a prior condition to receipt to payment for Hospital services, Hospital shall submit to Plan a standard detailed bill for such services within 60 days of the date of service, together with standard forms, discharge diagnoses and an Emergency Room treatment form if services were provided through the Emergency Room. Such detailed bill and related forms shall describe services provided by Hospital to Members with sufficient particularity to enable Plan to determine whether such services are Hospital Services. Payment of amounts owed by Plan to Hospital for Hospital Services shall be made by Plan to Hospital on or before the 30th calendar day following the date of Plan's receipt of a valid bill when prior authorisation for the service has been obtained from the Plan. A bill will be considered valid when it complies with all requirements of this subparagraph. Hospital may submit interim monthly bills for inpatient lengths of stay in excess of 30 days.

The same rules would typically apply for both day cases and outpatient services. The rates themselves would be shown separately and might be per diems, DRGs, DRG bands, a specially agreed per case contract rate for certain conditions or some combination of the above. Day cases would normally be payed on some form of value unit associated with the procedure code (similar to general practitioner fundholder's (GPFH) chargeable procedures). The majority of what the NHS categorizes as outpatient cases are seen in physicians' offices (typically adjoining the hospital or offsite) and are not seen as 'hospital activity'.

Formulae/rates for outliers and interhospital transfers are also likely to be included as appendices. The outlier ruling may be as simple as stating that any case with a total charge exceeding a set amount (say $80 000) will be reimbursed at 80% of the hospital's charges. Alternatively, the more complex Medicare based rules may be used or some other method of determination.

On this question of interhospital transfers this is an area that NHS contracts typically fail to deal with adequately. In the USA a formula for reimbursing the sending hospital may be used as follows:

DRG per case level of reimbursement/Medicare ALOS for the
DRG × actual LOS = sending hospital reimbursement

A further refinement would be to make the maximum amount reimbursable, some percentage of the DRG payment (say 80%). This would ensure amongst other things that the sending hospital does not make money by transferring cases. One way it could do this on the unmodified formula would be to have an actual LOS higher than the Medicare ALOS.

In the USA the receiving hospital might charge in the normal manner at the standard rate as if no transfer had taken place. A less generous reimbursement system would be to set a percentage of the normal payment once again, or have a similar formula to the sending hospital set in place.

A particularly important clause for managed care companies is something known as 'balance billing'. In most indemnity plans, hospitals and physicians 'balance bill' the patient for services which have not been approved as medically necessary or are not covered, thus shifting costs from the insurer to the patient and fuelling medical inflation. With the exception of the previously noted copayments a managed care contract would normally seek to prohibit this practice for authorized services, as it is regarded as a means of subverting utilization and cost controls. At the same time, it undermines a major selling-point and rationale of managed care – that health care costs become predictable and hence budgetable to the member.

The monies received from the plan would represent full and final payment for authorized services. If the service provided is not authorized the plan will not pay but the provider is permitted to pursue the claim directly with the member.

4 Grievances

This clause is notable for the fact that typically, the payor will require the hospital to inform it not only of the full particulars of any complaints it receives against the plan itself and its affiliated physicians, but also of any complaint by a member concerning any element of care in the hospital itself. The plan may in fact lead the investigation, requiring the hospital's full cooperation. Health authorities, by contrast, would normally take a much more hands-off approach on complaints about hospital care from their 'members'. Normally they would leave the hospital to conduct the investigation and the monitoring of complaints tends to consist only in receiving periodically very high-level summaries of all complaints received by each hospital. The details of the complaint, the content and findings of the investigation and the replies and actions taken are not normally seen, reflecting the new 'independence' of trusts. Perhaps this should be reviewed.

5 Hospital/plan relationship

This section acknowledges that the hospital acts as an independent contractor and is not an employee or agent of the plan. It is also likely to set the hospital's responsibilities in the coordination of benefits process.

6 Insurance and indemnification

This sets out the hospital's and plan's insurance and indemnification responsibilities including the policy and limits of reinsurance. In the malpractice atmosphere that US health care operates in, the existence of adequate insurance is an important issue.

7 Arbitration

Despite America's justified reputation for litigiousness, this section sets out an agreement to try and resolve disputes through an agreed arbitration process in the first instance – the use of the American Arbitration Association is a common route.

8 Terms of the agreement

This covers length of contract and the notice period. Typically contracts are renegotiated on an annual basis – although longer contract terms are relatively common – but the notice period for termination of services is much shorter than is normal in an NHS contract. 90 days would be common.

9 Miscellaneous

This covers a number of items such as what constitutes a formal communication, confidentiality, publicity restrictions, etc. One clause of potential interest to NHS purchasers and providers is the following:

> Plan and Hospital shall have access at reasonable times to the books, records and documents of Hospital and Plan relating to the provision of Hospital services, the cost thereof, the payments received by Hospital from members and the financial condition of Hospital; provided, however, Plan and Hospital

reimburse the other party for reasonable costs associated with making such documents available.

10 Location of services being delivered

This defines what services fall into which payment form, e.g. 'All cataracts will be reimbursed as a day case only'.

US physician contract

Some key features of physician contracts – both PCP and specialist – are set out below. There is some overlap with Appendix I – not surprisingly, given that these are also legal documents. Where the same categories are used, these are merely noted, to avoid repetition. Where an IPA model is in use, the contract will be between the IPA and the physician, rather than directly with the managed care company.

1 Definitions

This is the same as in Appendix I.

2 Obligations of practice

This sets out the terms on which the physician will operate within the plan. Of particular interest might be:

- claims. The same rules are likely to apply to physicians for claims (unless a capitation payment method is in operation) as for the hospitals, i.e. payment is dependent on a correctly documented claim within a defined period

- balance billing, as per hospital

- referrals and admissions. The physician has to agree to follow the managed care company's procedures for obtaining prior authorizations, etc.

- utilization management and quality assurance. This clause is important as the physician/practice will be required to cooperate with and participate in the utilization management, quality assurance, grievance, peer review, credentialling and recredentialling and audit procedures 'of the IPA, managed care contractors and payers and to comply with all final determinations rendered by such procedures'. This section may also include something along the following lines: 'Utilization review procedures shall include, but not be limited to, preadmission certification, concurrent and post-discharge review of covered person's hospital stays, avoidance of unnecessary duplicate tests and diagnostic procedures, and coordination of emergency services. In addition, the physician/ practice shall cooperate with IPA, Managed Care contractors and Payers in any on-site office and medical record reviews. Nothing in the above shall be deemed or construed to prohibit the physician/practice from making any recommendations to patients which are believed to be medically appropriate'

- contract terms. One-year contracts with termination clauses as per the hospital contracts are typical (i.e. 90 days' written notice from either party). Longer-term contracts are the subject of discussion as with the UK. As is also often the case in the NHS, whilst both parties are likely to state their desire for such agreements, shorter-term contracts remain dominant, because long-term contracts are considered too inflexible in a rapidly changing world.

3 Other clauses

These are similar to those in Appendix I: grievances, relationships, insurance, arbitration, reimbursement methods etc.

Appendix III

NHS contracts

In this appendix the principal features of a 'typical' NHS contract between a health authority and NHS trust are outlined. The author was heavily involved in the development of this particular documentation and is all too aware of its weaknesses and limitations. Because the internal market is a recent development with an emphasis initially on maintaining a 'steady state', contracts between purchasers and providers are still evolving. It is therefore dangerous to conclude that what is set out below is either 'typical' or 'desirable'. It certainly represents a compromise in parts. In presenting the thinking behind certain sections of the document, it will hopefully give a snapshot of the dynamics of NHS purchasing and the development of the market itself.

1 Parties to the contract

1.1   This agreement is between ... HEALTH AUTHORITY (the Purchaser) and the ... NHS TRUST (the Provider).

2 Objectives

2.1   The objective of this contract is to secure, for the residents of the ... provision of a defined level of health services to a defined quality standard for an agreed price.

3 Duration of the contract

3.1   This contract will apply for the financial year commencing 1st April 199...

Note that the 'standard' NHS contract is for one year. There are periodic calls for longer-term (3–5 years) contracts to be agreed, the rationale being that they will provide security and a framework for agreed change and that they will reduce the time spent on contract negotiation and paperwork. The principal obstacle to such a development is considered to be the annuality of NHS budget setting. This makes the 'security' of longer-term contracts often illusory. Volumes and prices are likely to be renegotiated each year (regardless of what the contract says) as government sets new targets, productivity requirements etc. and each party's financial position changes. For most providers the issue is less – Is purchaser X going to contract with me in two years' time? (often geography and clinical specialization make it a near inevitability) – but rather what will they pay us and how many cases will they require? For an organization which was once noted for its elaborate planning processes, the general inability to supply answers to these questions is stark.

4 Services to be provided

4.1   The services covered by this contract include:

Outpatients

All outpatient attendances at the Provider unit including the initial assessment and any subsequent outpatient consultations or treatment, associated diagnostic investigations and tests.

Inpatients and day cases

All emergency, urgent and elective inpatient and day case admissions and associated diagnostic and therapeutic services.

Accident and emergency services

The provision of a comprehensive 24-hour consultant-led accident and emergency service. This service should complement the primary care services and should meet those needs which are more appropriately met by a hospital-based service.

Day-care activity

Open-access services

Community services

4.1.1 Access to Services: Providers must take particular attention to ensure equity of access to generic health services for patients with disabilities, including those with a learning disability or mental illness.

4.1.2 Community Services must be, at a minimum, provided to the specification set out in Appendix ...

4.2   The following services are excluded from this contract:

    a) referrals made under the GP Fundholder Scheme by a GP Fundholder which are chargeable to the GP Fundholder

    b) specific waiting list initiatives, unless incorporated as an addendum to the contract

    c) tertiary referrals.

4.3   Detailed service specifications covering the services are those defined in Appendix ...

4.4   *Health gain specifications*. The Authority will continue to work with the provider in the development and monitoring of health gain specifications. Detailed service specifications covering the services are those defined in Appendix .... The specifications, which are supplementary to baseline contracts outline the requirements of the Purchaser for the services described and form the basis for service enquiry. A service enquiry will enable the purchaser to establish the baseline position for current service delivery by evaluating the appropriateness and quality of service and identifying any deficiencies present. This process of making existing service delivery more explicitly linked with the monitoring process of health gain specifications will enable the Purchaser and the Provider to implement Local Strategies for Health. Providers will need to review services against these specifications and may need to vary service delivery to comply with these specifications. These specifications are not expected to give rise to any additional resource implications since they are seen to reflect current practice. Any proposed changes which are deemed necessary and which the provider feels will give rise to additional costs must receive prior agreement from the Purchaser. The health gain areas and service targets chosen are as follows:

- maternal and early child health   (breast-feeding initiative, vaccination and immunization)

- cardiovascular diseases   (assessment, diagnosis and
                                        early treatment)

- acute myocardial infarction   (basic CPR training for health
                                        care staff)

- respiratory diseases   (asthma standards)

- physical and sensory disabilities   (diabetes)

- osteoarthritis of the hip and
  knee

- acute myocardial infarction   (extended protocol)

- diabetes.

This section refers to the Welsh Office inspired initiative of moving towards 'contracting for health gain' with health gain being broadly interpreted as better outcomes/increased patient satisfaction. The difficulty in implementing the initiative centred around the time consuming nature of any monitoring, professional antipathy to some of the targets and the process itself, and the apparent greater priority given by central government and its agents to waiting-lists, waiting times and financial control.

4.5   *Clinical effectiveness.* The provider must be able to demonstrate that, where practicable, current practice is based on sound evidence of effectiveness. In addition, they must have in place systems to enable practitioners to acquire the skills to use such evidence, and to audit new developments.

The issue, once again, is how a purchaser monitors this and what is done if it becomes apparent that current practice is not based on sound evidence of effectiveness, where such evidence exists – the paucity of which is probably the greatest problem of all.

5 Facilities to be provided

5.1   Pursuant to the main terms of this agreement, the Provider shall provide the following facilities:

- accident and emergency services

- outpatient consulting rooms and treatment rooms

- major and minor theatre facilities

- intensive care/high-dependency facilities

- diagnostic services

- professional, technical and therapeutic services

- pharmaceutical services

- hotel services

- community services.

To be consistent with the needs of the contract at a standard equivalent to or approved by approved National Accreditation Boards, where appropriate.

6 Volume

Note the emphasis placed on volumes and contract pacing in contrast to the USA documentation.

6.1   The expected volume and mix of activity to be provided under this service agreement is set out in Appendix .... The Purchaser may, in agreement with the Provider, for the duration of the contract vary the volume and mix of activity. Such variation shall be within the contract sum, using applicable specialty tariffs.

6.2   The Provider, in agreement with the Purchaser, is required to draw up a PROFILE of projected monthly activity to achieve the annual contracted levels detailed in Appendix .... The Provider is required to pace contracts in line with the profile to ensure that all urgent and emergency cases are accommodated within the contract levels. The profile should take into account seasonal/historical variations in activity over the contract period. Any balance remaining will thus form the level of elective cases to be undertaken by the Provider. The balance of elective cases should be directed towards the achievement of the Patient's Charter and Total Waiting Times guarantees. Any increase in activity against the profiled monthly activity and above the agreed tolerance levels, must be discussed with the Purchaser during the following month. The profile may be revised by agreement with the Purchaser. Increases in activity over and above contract levels that have not been agreed in advance will not be funded. Although the effect on waiting lists will be monitored through the contract monitoring process, the onus is clearly with providers to notify the Purchaser in advance of any large increases in the waiting lists as a result of a change in referral patterns during the year.

6.3   DRG-based contracts will also be in place in shadow form during 199.../.... The provider will be required to produce monthly activity data by DRG for monitoring purposes.

This clause is in anticipation of the move to case-mix based contracting. The difficulties in promoting such an initiative are discussed in the main text.

6.4   Variances between anticipated and actual activity will be reviewed as part of the contract monitoring process.

7 Price

7.1   The contract price for work undertaken in respect of ... residents is detailed in Appendix ....

7.2   The contract sum includes an allowance for anticipated overall level of pay and price increases.

7.3   There will be no further adjustment regardless of whether there are any increases or decreases in the level of pay or prices.

7.4   The Provider will not give other Purchasers (including GP Fund-holders) more favourable treatment in respect of either prices, quality or access to services than those offered to the Purchaser. This does not prevent the Provider from offering surplus capacity to Purchasers nor should it be seen as precluding the purchase of higher quality services at a higher price.

This 'most favoured nation' clause is undermined by the lack of an independent audit of compliance. Providers rarely make public to Health Authorities the prices other purchasers are paying. In theory, the doctrine of no cross-subsidization should mean no price differentials exist. In practice, this is often not the case. Furthermore, Health Authorities are reluctant to enforce their own contracts on the grounds that to do so will put the NHS Trust into difficulties, which in turn rebounds on the Health Authority. This political and economic symbiosis between purchaser and provider is probably the single biggest reason the post-reform NHS remains in 'gridlock'.

7.5   The total contract sum will remain fixed providing that total weighted activity (i.e. cost per specialty case multiplied by activity) does not vary by more than 1% of the total inpatient, day case and outpatient contract sum.

7.6   Where the Provider performs in excess of contract activity, and this excess activity is agreed to in advance by the Purchaser, the Provider will be reimbursed at the rate of 25% marginal cost for both elective cases and emergency cases. (In each case the % marginal cost relates to the relevant specialty tariff.)

7.7   Where the Provider performs at less than contract activity, then the Provider will rebate the Purchaser against the contract sum as follows:

* for activity between 1% and 3% below contracted activity, 25% marginal cost

* for activity between 3% and 5% below contracted activity, 40% of standard tariff

* for activity over 5% below contracted activity, 50% of standard tariff.

During contract negotiations the actual percentages for tolerances, marginal costs and rebates may well change.

7.8   Intensive Treatment Unit (ITU) and other High-Cost cases. If the Provider sets any element of its tariff based on bed days for ITU/High-Cost cases, the Authority will pay a marginal rate of 50% up to a limit of £60 000 per individual case.

This is the Health Authority's attempt to create a 'stop-loss' provision. It often encounters considerable resistance from providers.

8 Invoicing and settlement

8.1   The Purchaser agrees to pay one twelfth of the contract price on the 16th day of each month subject to the provision of specified monitoring information – See Section 9 – Monitoring and Compliance.

8.2   Adjustments to the contract sum shall be agreed between the Purchaser and the Provider as and when required.

9 Monitoring and compliance

9.1   The Provider is required to maintain systems which will produce information to enable activity levels and quality standards to be monitored. The Provider undertakes to provide the Purchaser with the following information on the residents of ...

9.2   *Workload (monthly)*. This consists of:

- total, new and outpatient reattendances by specialty

- total completed inpatient and day case episodes by specialty with a sub analysis showing details of the number of elective and emergency admissions and the associated length of stay. A comparison of activity on a quarterly basis comparing activity in Provider Spells. Welsh Office definitions must be adhered to

- a contracting minimum data set (CMDS) will need to be completed for each episode of care. All inpatient activity should be procedure and DRG coded. The Provider will be responsible for discussing and agreeing developments in the coding and classification of inpatient episodes, daycases and outpatient data with the Purchaser. The CMDS must be provided in the agreed format by no later than six weeks after the month when the patient episode occurred. The Provider must supply a monthly extract containing contracting minimum data sets by 20th of each month. Failure to supply the extract within the deadline set will result in a £200 penalty being levied per working day. Where the Authority is the Major Purchaser of Services it must receive a PEDW Extract for all residents within its administrative boundaries regardless of Purchaser (i.e. including GPFH and Private Patients).

General

All patient activity (inpatients, day cases and outpatients) must be *GP coded* since all chargeable activity to GP Fundholders no longer forms part of the contract with ... Health Authority.

The Provider should ensure that systems are in place to identify all chargeable activity including diagnostic and paramedical services by current and potential GP fundholders.

Waiting-list information is required in the revised PPO1(W) format on a *monthly* basis by 21st of each month.

Total outpatient and new outpatient activity is required in accordance with the revised format of the Welsh Office PPO1(A) contract monitoring return on a monthly basis by no later than 21st of each month.

Total, new and repeat accident and emergency attendances.

Failure to supply PPO1s by the due date will result in a £200 penalty being levied per working day.

Activity relating to community services is required as stipulated in the minimum data set of the community services specification and also the Welsh Office procurement monitoring return for community services activity (PPO2) and High Level Performance Indicators. These returns may be amended in line with national requirements.

Total number of GP Pathology and Radiology open access tests by GP Practice and by test type or Welcan Units.

In order to provide the above information on each episode of care, the provider will record all attendances and ensure they are post-coded and GP coded.

10 Quality

Statement of intent

10.1   Quality specifications are subject to continuous review (primarily via the Quality Fora). The standards listed below represent current requirements and are subject to change based on mutual consent. The existence of these standards within the contract *does not* preclude the adoption of new or refined standards or their adoption within the contract in year where both parties are in agreement to this.

10.2   Notwithstanding the specific quality standards detailed in this document, the Provider will be expected to provide services to a standard:

10.2.1 that may reasonably be expected to fall within the definition of good UK practice

10.2.2 that meets locally agreed clinical protocols

10.2.3 that meets locally agreed service/Health Gain specifications.

10.3   The Provider will be required to comply with all relevant legislation. Where compliance is not currently achieved, Providers should give details, in their Operational Plan, of their corrective programme. Progress reports should be provided to the Purchaser at six-monthly intervals. The existence of Crown Immunity should not prevent the Provider behaving as if any piece of relevant legislation did apply.

10.4   A copy of the Provider's High Level Indicators Report (Secondary Care and Community Health Services) is required for each quarter in line with Welsh Office deadlines. Failure to supply HLIs by the due date will result in a £200 penalty per working day.

10.5   Patients should not be admitted on a Friday for an elective procedure scheduled for Monday. This will be monitored via the CMDS and for each case a financial penalty of £300 will be levied. However, no penalty will be imposed before the Provider is given the opportunity to investigate and provide an explanation.

10.6   The Provider must maintain an incident record of partial and total hospital closures, together with reasons for such occurrences. Legitimate reasons for partial/full closures include:

- abnormal emergency admission rates
- ward closures as a result of infection
- hospital closure because of emergency admissions redirected as a result of another Provider's closure.

The Provider must keep a record of the midnight bed state. Where the Provider is unable to demonstrate a legitimate reason for either partial or full closure, a £2000 financial penalty will be levied on each occasion.

10.7   The Provider is expected to achieve a specialty reattendance ratio as identified at Appendix ... (New:total outpatient attendances) or less. The Provider must be able to demonstrate that there has been a reduction in attendance ratios in specialties from 1995/6 levels, unless otherwise agreed with the Purchaser that the current ratios represent optimum clinical practice.

10.8   Provider will maintain a documented system for the recording of untoward incidents, which includes definitions, procedures and action taken. A summary of untoward incidents and action taken are to be supplied every six months (September/March).

10.9   The Provider will provide to the Purchaser within one month of signing this agreement, details of the procedures in place and definitions used relating to untoward incidents.

10.10 The Provider is required to have in place an agreed and regular programme of validation for inpatient and outpatient waiting-lists.

10.11 The Provider will work towards ensuring systems are developed to provide information to the Purchaser on referral rates by specialty to enable the analysis of the relationship between referral rates, activity undertaken and waiting-times by specialty and consultant.

10.12 The Provider is also expected to adhere to DGM(92)102 (*Competing for Quality*) and ensure that further development of market testing of support services is undertaken and achieves greater efficiencies and value for money.

11 Local quality standards

The standards below were constructed from issues considered to be of importance to local people and GPs. Most providers dislike any contract clauses that incorporate financial penalties arguing that it's all stick and no carrot. Monitoring some of the clauses can be problematic as it requires the active cooperation of GPs. The objective is uniform reporting but this is difficult to achieve, as those GPs who feel strongly about the standards and/or perceive a problem in that area report failures, whilst others might not.

11.1 In 199.../... a number of quantifiable quality targets have been set for local standards which will have financial implications for compliance/non-compliance. The sum of £14 000 will be held in reserve on the entire contract sum. This sum will be paid in quarterly instalments of £3500 where the Provider meets the standard set below. Successful Providers will also receive as a bonus a percentage of monies equivalent to their share of ... Health Authority's total contract allocation held back from Providers who fail to meet set standards. The quality standards for which the above applies are as follows:

- notification of death to GP within 24 hours, 100%

- discharge summary within 2 working days, 95%

- discharge letter within 2 weeks, 95%.

The content of summaries and monitoring processes will be subject to negotiation. It is envisaged that GPs will inform the Purchaser of non-compliance. No penalties will be levied before the Provider has been given the opportunity to investigate and provide an explanation.

11.2 Failure to provide a reply by the Chief Executive within four working weeks of receiving a complaint will result in a £100 penalty being imposed per working day in excess of deadline. The Provider will supply monitoring information as part of Quarterly High Level Indicator Reports.

11.3 Failure to admit a patient onto the next available list following a second cancelled operation (where the reason for cancellation lies with the Provider) – £500 on each occasion.

11.4 New outpatient attendances must result in the production of a clinical letter to the referring GP within 14 working days. Monitoring will be on an exception basis by GPs to the Commissioning Authority. Where the standard is not met on more than 100 occasions across all practices in a year, the Provider will automatically forfeit the £14 000 quality reserve monies.

11.5 Patients must be seen by the Consultant or Registrar at first outpatient attendance. Where another member of the firm writes the clinical letter it must state whether the Consultant or Registrar has been consulted.

11.6 Any treatment undertaken within 21 days of an outpatient or day case procedure, occurring as a result of a complication from the aforementioned procedure, will only be paid at 25% of the relevant specialty tariff. (Up to 4% of the total day case volume for that specialty. Above 3% no payment will be made.) Monitoring will be via CMDS. No adjustment will be made before the Provider is given the opportunity to investigate and provide an explanation for the case in question.

11.7 An unplanned inpatient readmission following associated elective admission occurring within 30 days of discharge will be paid at 25% of the relevant specialty tariff (up to 4% of the total inpatient volume for that specialty; above 4% no payment will be made) for the following specialties:

- ophthalmology
- ENT.

Monitoring will be via CMDS. No adjustment will be made before the Provider is given an opportunity to investigate and provide an explanation for the case in question.

12 Hospital closure

The Provider is required to ensure a documented bed management policy is in place and to provide a copy to the Authority annually. This policy must include specific instructions guarding against ring-fencing arrangements or protectionism of beds for elective treatments at the expense of emergency admissions (see also 10.6).

13 Systems

The Provider will be required to develop and maintain the following systems aimed at ensuring patient safety and prognosis:

13.1   a system of medical audit recognized by the Purchaser's Director of Public Health Medicine. A selection of audit topics will be undertaken as a result of discussion with the DPHM with the results made available to the Authority in conjunction with the Authority Independent Medical Adviser

13.2   a system of nursing audit recognized by the Purchaser's Director of Public Health Nursing

13.3   evidence that the Provider is working towards a multidisciplinary system of clinical audit

13.4   systems for the audit of professional, technical, diagnostic and therapeutic services (NB to be developed if not in place)

13.5   trust will provide details of system and definitions, and will maintain a documented system for the recording of untoward incidents, which includes definitions, procedures and action taken. A summary of untoward incidents and action taken are to be supplied every six months (September/March)

13.6   a Drugs and Therapeutic Committee which, as part of its remit, deals with the promotion of rational prescribing, taking total costs to the NHS into account. It should also promote means of ensuring compliance, e.g. agreed formulary

13.7   a system for the establishment of written Shared Care Management/prescribing protocols which define the responsibilities of GPs and Consultants in instances where patients could experience continuity of care problems after discharge (as outlined in WHC(91)94)

13.8   a system for the audit of pharmaceutical services against standards in *Standards for Pharmaceutical Services in Provider Units in*

Wales issued by Welsh Office under DGM(93)119 and the provision of an annual exception report of compliance with the standards to be sent to the Purchaser

13.9   the Provider must adhere to the minimum prescribing requirements stipulated in the Welsh Office circular WHC(91)94. The resource implications associated with this change in policy are within the funded contract price

13.10 the Provider is required to have agreed its Major Incident Plan with the Purchaser in accordance with the requirements of WHC(94)148. The Provider is required to send a copy of this plan to the Director of Public Health at ... Health Authority within one month of the date at which the contract is signed

13.11 the Provider is required to maintain the following systems designed to improve and assess non-clinical aspects of the service:

- patient surveys

- a patient's handbook (updated appropriately)

- a system for patients to make complaints and suggestions, which is well publicized and adhered to by staff

- the production of guidance handouts to support discharge

13.12 the Provider must be able to demonstrate that it has an adequate system in place both for public/staff security and asset control. Security will be assessed against relevant Welsh Office advice and circulars including DGM(94)85 and the Allitt Report.

14 Patient's Charter waiting times guarantees

Appendix ... details the Patient's Charter rights and standards which providers are required to adhere to. Set out below are those areas where financial penalties are to be levied where the Provider fails to comply with these standards.

14.1   All providers are expected to achieve the Patient's Charter guarantees and Caring for the Future targets including the following:

- no patients waiting more than one month for urgent treatment

- no patients waiting more than two years for non-urgent treatment

- no patients waiting over 18 months for a hip, knee and cataract procedure.

Within the combined contracted activity shown at Appendix C and agreed waiting-list initiative activity it is implicit that the Provider will ensure that patients will be treated within the time limits set by the Patient's Charter. Failure to treat patients within the Patient's Charter one month, 18 months and two years targets as appropriate, will result in the imposition of a penalty equivalent to 125% of the relevant speciality tariff. Further, failure to notify the Purchaser of patients waiting for three weeks in the case of urgent treatment, or those within three months or less of the other waiting-times targets, including the absence of a firm admission date, will result in a penalty equivalent to 75% of the relevant specialty cost of care. The Total Waiting-Time Guarantees come into operation from 1st April 1995. All cases referred from 1st April 1995 will be covered by the guarantee. The Authority has set the following standard: no patient referred after 1st April 1995 will wait longer than six months for a New Outpatient appointment. Failure to treat patients within this time period will result in the imposition of a penalty equivalent to 300% of the relevant specialty tariff for New Outpatient treatment. The application of these penalties shall be waived if, in the opinion of the Purchaser:

- the Provider can demonstrate that they have satisfactorily addressed the problem

- the breach of Patient's Charter targets is the consequence of exceptional circumstances, e.g. Hospital closure due to infection or exceptional emergency caseload

- if it can be demonstrated that the Purchaser has contracted for insufficient volumes to enable Patient's Charter guarantees to be met.

The Provider will work with the Purchaser in moving towards new guarantees or targets as they are announced by the Welsh Office.

15 Care in the community

15.1   The Provider will be required to adhere to WHC(90)1 and WHC(95)7 and the Purchaser's protocol regarding both the

discharge arrangements of patients from hospital-based ac-
commodation and the arrangements for those patients requiring
health care services who are already in a community setting. A
protocol has been agreed on a Joint Agency basis with Social
Services in respect of the new arrangements for Care in the
Community, particularly addressing the issue of joint assessments
for health and social care needs:

- local discharge arrangements should reflect the needs and wishes
  of the patient, wherever possible. Patients should only be discharged after adequate arrangements have been made for their
  continuing care

- the Providers must ensure that where discharge to a nursing/
  residential home takes place patients and/or their relatives
  should sign a document stating that they have been made aware
  of the financial consequences of the action being taken.

15.2   Patients being transferred from Hospital care needing specialized
       'hi-tech' health care at home for conditions and/or treatments
       specified in FHSL(W)13/95, shall have in place a written shared
       care agreement between the consultant and GP prior to discharge.
       A contract with an appropriate provider for the supply of relevant
       care shall also be in place prior to discharge.

16 Compliance visits

16.1   The Purchaser reserves the right to visit and check that the
       Provider is complying with any or all aspects of the contract. This
       includes services subcontracted to other organizations which form
       part of this contract. The visit may include Authority Directors, GP
       Forum or CHC members. Notice will be given of a visit but the
       Purchaser reserves the right to visit without notice. In the latter
       event however, the Chief Executive of the Provider will be advised
       upon arrival. The Trust should ensure any relevant subcontracted
       organizations are aware of this arrangement. Following a
       compliance visit or other noting of apparent non-performance, the
       findings will be discussed with the Provider and corrective action
       agreed and taken as necessary.

17 Tertiary referrals

17.1   Emergency tertiary referrals will not require prior approval providing the referral has been initiated by a consultant. However, the Provider is required to inform the Purchaser of which Provider will receive the referral at the time of referral. In determining where to refer, Consultants should pay due regard to where the Purchaser has negotiated contracts. Consultants should not refer patients to other Consultants for elective procedures which they would normally carry out themselves.

17.2   The Provider will be expected to seek prior authorization from the Purchaser in accordance with an agreed protocol before any non-emergency tertiary referrals are initiated.

18 Transfer and subcontracting

18.1   The Provider will not subcontract any part of the services covered by this contract unless prior agreement is reached.

18.2   Providers will ensure that where the services of practitioners of the professions supplementary to medicine are subcontracted by the Trust, such services must be provided by state registered practioners.

19 Changes in clinical practice/medical science

19.1   It is essential that Providers assess the implications of any proposed service changes in terms of both the quality and cost of care prior to these changes taking place. Proposed changes which either affect the number of patients treated or which the Provider feels will give rise to additional costs must be agreed prior to the development/change taking place. Any claims for additional funding arising after a particular change/development has commenced will not be considered.

19.2   The Provider will not seek funding for any scheme from Welsh Office which will have implications for the contract without prior discussion and agreement of the Authority.

19.3   The Provider must demonstrate a willingness to work with the Purchaser in commissioning, managing and carrying out research to promote beneficial changes in services. This research must be conducted ethically, to high standards, and with full knowledge and consent of patients and other participants.

20 Management of waiting-lists

20.1   The Provider is responsible for managing all waiting-lists on behalf of the Purchaser although ownership clearly lies with the Purchasing Authority. The Authority regards the management of waiting-lists as a key priority for 199 ... and the Provider will be expected to adopt the requirements specified by the Authority in developing this process.

20.2   The Provider may, under the terms of the contract, be required to select patients under given criteria for referral to either the Treatment centres or other Provider units following the award of a waiting-list initiative. The following key requirements should be addressed:

- to ensure that all waiting-list data are coded by procedure and/or condition to enable the prompt and accurate analysis of waiting-lists

- all waiting-lists should be priority coded, i.e. Urgent, Soon and Routine. The Provider will discuss the development of further classifications for management purposes with the Purchaser. The Provider will ensure that the waiting-lists for GPFH chargeable procedures/attendances made by GP Fundholders are clearly separated from the Purchaser's waiting-lists.

- separate waiting-lists should be maintained for inpatients and day cases for all specialties

- the Provider must have in place a demonstrable system of waiting-list validation and management and identification of patients. At a minimum this system must cover the tasks set out in Appendix .... The Provider must be able to produce an audit trail of actions taken as per Appendix .... If the Authority on examination of the waiting-list system is not satisfied that adequate validation and management has/is taking place, it reserves the right to: (i) carry out a validation exercise and (ii) if necessary, offer patients alternative Providers for their treatment. Where such an exercise, has to be undertaken, the Authority will: (i) charge for the Authority's staff time taken and deduct this directly from the contract sum, and (ii) deduct £300 from the contract sum for every patient who has already had the operation, was clinically unsuitable, or refused alternative centre for treatment, deferred yet not identified as such in relation to Patient's Charter, (iii) where Patient's Charter breaches result from inadequate validation/management of the waiting-list, the Authority will deduct any cost of treating these cases at alternative centres from the contract sum in addition to the above.

20.3   The Provider will ensure that where the waiting-list of a consultant within the Provider unit is such that Total Waiting-Time Guarantees cannot be met, then:

- the Purchaser will be advised of the situation

- following discussion with the Purchaser, the waiting-list for that consultant will be closed, and no new referrals will be accepted until the waiting-list has been reduced to be within the Total Waiting-Time Guarantee, unless the patient is aware of the waiting time and chooses to go onto the waiting-list in the full knowledge that the Total Waiting-Times Guarantees will not apply.

20.4   The Provider will ensure that information systems are adopted and used in such a way that the waiting-lists are managed in accordance with DGM(94)134 or later relevant Welsh Office guidance.

20.5   Treatment Centres. The Provider may opt for the Authority to take responsibility for contacting GPs/patients concerning the possibility of a Treatment Centre placement/alternative Provider. The Purchaser would subsequently inform the Provider which cases remain on its waiting-list and their Charter status. Should this option be taken, the Provider must submit the relevant patient details from waiting-lists for the relevant specialties at not less than monthly intervals for the attention of the Director of Public Health.

21 Variation of contract terms

21.1   There may be circumstances during the year which will prevent the full discharge of the agreement through no fault of either party. Circumstances where this may occur might include:

- significant changes in case mix of the anticipated workload

- changes in medical science and medical practice which may affect the cost and the type of cases that can be treated

- major incidents, extreme weather conditions, epidemics or other 'force majeure' occurrences.

The effect of these factors on contract activity and sum should be discussed at the earliest opportunity in order that appropriate adjustments may be agreed to the satisfaction of both parties.

21.2   The need for any variation should be discussed at the earliest opportunity and any variation will be made with the full consent of both parties.

22   Remedies for non-performance

22.1   In the event of the Provider or the Purchaser not performing according to the agreed terms of the service agreement, the following procedure shall apply:

- where one party considers that the other party has under performed its contractual obligations, that party will instigate a meeting with the other within 14 days

- following the meeting, the party which has not performed adequately will be given a specified time to resolve the issue

- where non-performance has not been rectified within the agreed timescale the other party will have the right to refer to arbitration.

23   Audit requirements

23.1   The Provider will be required to achieve NHS minimum audit standards including value for money, probity and systems audit in respect of all services provided under this contract. The Purchaser will have access to the recommendations and management action arising from Audit Commission reports. The Director of Finance of the Authority and of the Provider Unit will agree suitable monitoring arrangements to ensure compliance by the provider in this respect. If the NHS minimum audit standards are not being achieved this shall be notified promptly to the Director of Finance of the Authority. The Authority's Director of Finance may require further information in respect of cost, price and operation of this contract in order to gain an understanding of any variances to the contract.

23.2 The Provider shall comply with their own Standing Orders, Standing Financial Instructions (including Procedure Notes) and Personnel Policies.

24 Confidentiality

24.1 Both parties will ensure that the confidentiality of the patient and their records is upheld at all times.

25 General practitioner direct access to services

25.1 *Procedures.* General Practitioners must be afforded the option of direct access to procedures and waiting-lists where a protocol has been agreed. The priority for protocol production should be agreed between Provider and local General Practitioners. The principal means of agreeing prioritization and the method of protocol production should be via the DMC and the Local General Practitioner Forum. Before a protocol is implemented, any financial consequences will need to be agreed with the Purchaser.

26 Service changes and fair purchasing

Providers must comply with DGM(95)17 *Fair Purchasing* and ... Health Authority's *Protocol for Dealing with Provider Initiated Competitive Service Developments* (Appendix ...).

27 Arbitration and conciliation

27.1 In the event of a dispute over non-performance arising between the Purchaser and the Provider Unit in relation to this Contract and which cannot be agreed by both parties, the issue, as a final resort, shall be resolved by arbitration.

27.2 The dispute shall (unless the parties concur on the appointment of an alternative arbitrator) be referred to the Welsh Office arbitration procedures.

28 Authorization

For and on behalf of the ... HEALTH AUTHORITY

Signature   Date

....

....

For and on behalf of the ... NHS TRUST

Signature   Date

....

....

HMO benefit packages

The following are exclusions and limitations on covered benefits detailed in a members' booklet. They are set out below as they give a reasonable indication of the restrictions which might apply to HMO members (depending on their benefit package).

1. Acupuncture.

2. Biofeedback.

3. Blood or blood plasma and the cost of securing the services of blood donors.

4. Circumcision for non-medically indicated reasons after one month of age.

5. Any cosmetic surgery or any hospital, physician, or other health service related thereto, except to the extent medically necessary to restore function. Reconstructive surgery is not covered unless such service follows trauma which causes anatomic functional impairment and if such trauma occurred on or after the effective date of the member's coverage or is needed to correct a congenital disease or anomaly which has resulted in a functional defect. However, reconstructive mammoplasty following mastectomy is a covered benefit.

6. Complications resulting from cosmetic and/or experimental procedures.

7. Consultations and/or office visits for the purpose of obtaining cosmetic and/or experimental procedures.

8. Coverage for a newborn or other child of a dependent child.

9. Custodial, domiciliary care, rest cures, or any examination and/or care ordered by a court of law which has not received prior authorization by a primary care physician, approved by the Plan and arranged through, or provided at, a participating Plan facility.

10. Dentistry

- restorative services and supplies necessary to repair or replace sound natural teeth are not covered, even if loss is due to an injury or accident

- oral surgery (unless necessary due to an injury or accident involving the jaw or any bone structure adjoining the jaw which occurs while the member is enrolled in the Plan and for which immediate treatment is requested by the member within 48 hours of the accidental injury, or unless necessary for conditions such as fractures or malignant tumors of the jawbone) which is part of an orthodontic treatment program, or which is required for correction of an occlusal defect, or which encompasses orthognathic surgical procedures

- dental services performed in a hospital or any outpatient care facility and any related fees.

11. Except in event of emergency any services or supplies that were not authorized and/or arranged by a primary care physician or the Plan. Services for pregnancy and/or delivery outside the service area on or beyond the 35th week of gestation are excluded.

12. Expenses incurred for an illness or injury suffered in connection with the commitment of or intent to commit a felony.

13. Experimental medical, surgical or other experimental health care procedures, services or supplies. Experimental procedures, services or supplies are those which, in the judgment of the Plan: (a) are in a testing stage or in field trials on animals or humans; (b) do not have required final federal regulatory approval for commercial distribution for the specific indications and methods of use assessed; (c) are not in accordance with generally accepted standards of medical practice; or (d) have not yet been shown to be consistently effective for the diagnosis or treatment of the member's condition.

14. Eye surgery (radial keratotomy) to correct refraction errors.

15. Routine foot care such as removal of corns or callouses, the trimming of nails, the treatment of tarsalgia, metatarsalgia or bunion, except for the operation which involves the exposure of bones, tendons, or ligaments.

16. Hearing aids, eyeglasses or contact lenses or the fitting thereof, except for the first pair of lenses (this may include contact lens, or placement of intraocular lens or eyeglass lens only) following a cataract operation.

17. Immunizations as related to foreign travel and/or employment.

18. The cost of services which are covered through a group insurance mechanism or governmental program, such as workers' compensation, occupational disease laws and other employers' liability laws. Should a member have the cost of services denied by one of the above insurance programs, the Plan will only consider payment of covered services in those cases where the member received services in accordance with the Plan's referral procedures. The Plan will not cover the cost of services that were denied by the above insurance programs for failure to meet administrative or filing requirements.

19. Intrauterine devices.

20. Care for military service-connected disabilities and conditions for which the member is legally entitled to services and for which facilities are reasonably accessible to the member.

21. All services and drugs in connection with obesity, including surgical procedures such as gastric bypass, gastric stapling, and any other procedures and experimental services specifically used for treatment of obesity, except other services, programs and treatments within standard medical practice policies and which are authorized and approved by the Plan.

22. Foot orthotics, i.e. custom shoes, custom inserts for shoes or boots.

23. Personal comfort items which shall include but not be limited to telephones, televisions, extra meal trays, and personal hygiene items.

24. Physical examinations for employment, insurance, or recreational activities.

25. Prescription drugs unless provided as a covered benefit.

26. Private duty nursing in the hospital or in the home is excluded except when ordered by the attending physician and approved by the Plan for medically necessary reasons.

27. Provider's clerical charges for no-shows, telephone calls, completion of forms, transfer of medical records, generation of correspondence to other parties, etc.

28. Psychiatric or psychological examinations, testing, or treatments for purposes of obtaining or maintaining employment or insurance or relating to judicial or administrative proceedings.

29. Remedial education, including services which are extended beyond the period necessary for evaluation and diagnosis of learning and behavioral disabilities or for mental retardation or autism disabilities.

30. School physicals (covered only when member has not previously had a physical with his or her primary care physician during the contract year).

31. Sex change operations, reversal of voluntary sterilization, infertility service required because of such reversal, in vitro fertilization programs, and the GIFT program.

32. Treatment for smoking cessation.

33. Spinal manipulation which shall mean the detection, treatment and correction of structural imbalance, subluxation or misalignment of the vertebral column in the human body, for the purpose of alleviating pressure on the spinal nerves and its associated effects related to such structural imbalance, misalignment or distortion, by physical or mechanical means.

34. Services and supplies provided in connection with any organ or bone marrow transplants except for the following list of non-experimental procedures when authorized by the Plan and meeting Plan criteria: heart, kidney, lung, corneal and liver transplants, bone marrow transplants for leukemia, Hodgkin's disease, non-Hodgkin's lymphoma, severe combined immunodeficiency disease, aplastic anemia and Wiscott–Aldridge syndrome. At the discretion of the Plan, this list may be amended from time to time in accordance with accepted medical and community standards. Charges associated with obtaining donor organs are excluded unless both donor and recipient are Plan members.

35. Artificial or mechanical heart expenses.

36. Therapy due to an injury will be covered only to the extent of restoration to the pre-trauma level. Speech Therapy will be covered only to the extent of restoration to the level of the pre-trauma, pre-illness, or pre-condition speech function.

37. Travel and transportation are excluded except for medically necessary and ambulance services which must be approved and authorized by the Plan.

38. Orthoptics or vision/visual training and any associated supplemental testing.

39. Failure to comply with recommended treatment is an option for a member. In such cases, the Plan will assume no further liability for the

particular condition unless the member later decides to follow prescribed treatment under the care of the ordering physician and subject to the terms of the Evidence of Coverage.

40. Any service, supplies or treatment not specifically covered in this Evidence of Coverage and any other procedure determined not to be medically necessary.

41. Any eye examination, or any corrective eyewear, required by an employer as a condition of employment.

42. Services for pregnancy or a pregnancy-related condition provided to dependent children on non-federally qualified products, unless covered under a Rider and shown as a covered benefit.

Table IV.1: Illustrative example of benefits in a health plan

Services	Annual deductibles	Comments
Physician's services		
PCP office visit	$10 copay, then covered at 100%	Referral form required
Specialist office visit	$15 copay, then covered at 100%	
Preventive care	$10 copay per visit, then covered at 100%	Includes periodic check-ups, well-baby care, annual GYN exam, lab. and X-ray services, and vision and hearing screenings for children up to age 18
Maternity care	$100 copay per pregnancy, then covered at 100%	Includes all pre- and post-natal out-patient care for subscriber or spouse only. Dependent child maternity care is not covered
Out-of-hospital lab., X-ray, and other diagnostic services	Covered at 100%	Referral form required
Hospital services		
Inpatient care (includes physician in-hospital visits)	$250 copay per admission, then covered at 100%	Includes maternity care for subscriber or spouse only; dependent child maternity care is not covered. Coverage provided for unlimited days in a semi-private room
Lab. and X-ray	Covered at 100%	In-hospital services only
Outpatient surgery/services (includes physician's fee for surgery)	$100 copay per admission, then covered at 100%	When medically necessary. Copay applies to any services which are provided in the outpatient surgery unit, except blood transfusions and chemotherapy
Inpatient surgery/services	Covered at 100%	When medically necessary

Table IV.1: *Continued*

Services	Annual deductibles	Comments
Emergency services (in or out of service area) (emergency care is retrospectively reviewed to determine medical necessity. Member may be responsible for charges related to visit)		
Emergency room (includes emergency care by a physician)	$50 copay, then covered at 100%	Copay waived if admitted
Urgent care center	$25 copay, then covered at 100%	Pre-authorization required
Ambulance	$25 copay each way, then covered at 100%	When medically necessary. Copay waived if admitted
Mental health care and substance abuse services (mental health care and substance abuse services are administered by Sentara Mental Health Management)		
Inpatient mental health care	$100 copay per day, then covered at 100%, up to a combined maximum (with Inpatient Substance Abuse Services) of 30 days per contract year. (Up to ten inpatient days may be converted to 20 partial days.)	
Inpatient substance abuse services	$150 copay per day, then covered at 100%, up to a combined maximum (with Inpatient Mental Health Care) of 30 days per contract year. (Up to ten inpatient days may be converted to 20 partial days.)	There is a 90-day lifetime maximum for substance abuse rehabilitation
Outpatient mental health care and substance abuse services	$35 copay per visit/hour, then covered at 100% up to 20 visits per contract year	

Table IV.1: *Continued*

Services	Annual deductibles	Comments
Other services		
Allergy injection	$5 copay per injection in addition to any applicable office visit copay, then covered at 100%	
Allergy serum	Not covered	
Allergy testing	$25 copay, then covered at 100%	Referral form required
Durable medical equipment	Covered at 100%, up to $1,000 per contract year	Pre-authorization required. Does not include replacement, repairs or duplicates
Intermittent home health care	Covered at 100%	Pre-authorization required. Following inpatient hospital care or in lieu of hospitalization
Infertility services	Covered at 50%	Referral form required. Counseling and testing as determined medically appropriate by the Plan
Orthopedic and prosthetic appliances	Initial surgically-implanted appliances covered at 100%. Non-surgically implanted appliances covered up to a combined limit of $1,000 per contract year	Replacement, repair and duplicates of prosthetic and orthopedic appliances are only covered as described in the Evidence of Coverage

Table IV.1: *Continued*

Services	Annual deductibles	Comments
Other services (*continued*) Preventive dental	$30 copay per visit, then covered at 100% for two visits per contract year which includes: ● oral examination ● routine cleaning ● bitewing X-rays (as necessary) ● fluoride treatment for children under age 18	There is a 20% discount off the Provider's Usual and Customary Charges for dental services and appliances. (The dental services and appliances discount is not a guaranteed benefit of the Plan's Evidence of Coverage)
Preventive vision	$5 copay for one exam every 24-months by a participating vision provider, then covered at 100%	There is a 20% discount off the provider's Usual and Customary Charges for vision materials and supplies. (The eyewear discount is not a guaranteed benefit of the Plan's Evidence of Coverage)
Skilled nursing facility care	$250 copay maximum per admission, then covered at 100%, up to 100 days per contract year. Maximum includes copays from any preceding hospital stays	Pre-authorization required. Following inpatient hospital care or in lieu of hospitalization
Therapy (short-term physical, occupational, speech and cardiac rehabilitation)	$15 copay per treatment/visit, then covered at 100%, up to 90 consecutive days lifetime per illness or condition	Pre-authorization required

Table IV.1: *Continued*

Services	Annual deductibles	Comments
Tubal ligation	$250 copay, in addition to applicable outpatient surgery or inpatient copay, then covered at 100%	Referral form required
Vasectomy	$100 copay, in addition to applicable outpatient surgery or inpatient copay, then covered at 100%	Referral form required
Other information Lifetime maximum		There is no lifetime dollar amount maximum
Out-of-pocket maximum per calendar year	$1500 maximum per individual; $3000 family maximum	Does not include copays for outpatient mental health or substance abuse rehabilitative service visits, dental, vision, tubal ligations, vasectomies, infertility services or any Ridered benefit copays
Waiting-period for preexisting conditions		None

Examples of Sentara's treatment authorization protocols

SUBJECT: Chronic Pain Management Program
COVERED: Program coverage is limited to one per lifetime
EXCEPTIONS: None
REFERRAL: Written referral not required; pre-certification by plan is required
Co-pay: Specialist office visit co-pay
POLICY: Chronic Pain Management is covered on a case by case basis under our case management program. OHP/SHP accept the financial liability for this program. The pain management program is contracted with Maryview Hospital Pain Center
OBJECTIVE: • identify cases appropriate for the chronic pain program
                • steer cases to appropriate level of care
                • eliminate unnecessary hospitalization and over-utilization

PROCEDURES:

The primary care physician or referring physician's office initiates call to Sentara ADS Medical Care Management Department and refers member to the coordinator. The coordinator will request that reason for referral has been documented in patient's chart.

The PCP or referring physician's office must supply the following information:

• member's name
• plan name and ID number
• fax copy of member's chart to the coordinator.

If referring physician is a specialist he/she checks with member's PCP to concur with treatment.

When information is received, cases will be reviewed by the co-ordinator and then referred to the medical director for review and approval. The physician's office will be contacted if more information is needed. Acceptance into the pain program is dependent on meeting the criteria (see Attachment I, Criteria).

As part of the preliminary assessment, an evaluation by the Sentara Mental Health Management Medical Director may be required at the request of the plan's Medical Director. During this evaluation process, alternative levels of care may be identified. If approved by Medical Director, the co-ordinator at Maryview Hospital Pain Center is contacted and given the following information:

- member's name
- member's ID
- diagnosis
- authorization number.

A summary and recommendations will be sent to the Medical Director and PCP. The Medical Director will then approve a treatment plan. An authorization letter will be issued to the Maryview Hospital Pain Center authorizing the treatment plan.

A copy of the authorization letter and treatment plan will be sent to the member's primary care physician.

The member calls and sets up an appointment at Maryview Hospital Pain Center for his/her program to begin.

If more time is needed in the program than originally stated, the Medical Director must pre-certify any extended days.

If initial assessment by the pain management consultant results in a recommendation for consultative care *other than* the formal pain management program (inpatient or outpatient), all subsequent care will require approval by PCP.

Attachment I: Chronic pain management

Patients referred for pain management will be approved by the plan and certified for a specific time period and/or services. Members referred may be identified by the plan and/or participating physicians; however, notification must be given to the primary care physician and he/she must be in agreement. All pertinent information will be reviewed including: medical records, claims profiles, drug utilization profiles, physician records, and physician referrals, etc.
Criteria:

- documentation of chronic pain (>6 months duration)
  - refractory to medical/surgical management

- which significantly limits normal functioning
- requires increasing medical services
- **and** documentation of failed attempts at management by PCP, specialist, and/or therapy providers, etc.
- **and** increasing utilization of medical services related to pain (ER/UCC, physician visits, pharmaceuticals, etc.)
- **and** patient not terminally ill
- **and** patient/family ready, willing and able to attend, participate and comply with the pain management treatment outlined by the program
- **or** documentation of drug dependence related to a chronic pain syndrome.

Criteria for inpatient pain treatment (prior to outpatient Chronic Pain Management Program):

- need for inpatient drug detoxification
- need for continuous observation of condition/functioning.

SUBJECT:	Screening for ovarian cancer
EXCEPTIONS:	Not covered for routine screening in asymptomatic individuals
REFERRAL:	Required for HMO specialist OV
Co-pay:	Appropriate OV co-pay or co-insurance
CPT CODES:	86316 (CA-125); 76830 (echography, transvaginal); 76856 (echography, pelvic non-obstetric)

PROCEDURE:

Screening for ovarian cancer is covered for members who have one first degree relative (i.e. mother, sister, or child) with a history of ovarian, breast, colon or endometrial cancer. The following services are covered if deemed medically necessary: pelvic examination, CA-125, transvaginal ultrasound, and/or pelvic ultrasound.

Note: For prophylactic oophorectomy, see medical policy Surgery – 33

Routine screening by abdominal or vaginal ultrasound or measurement of CA-125 levels in women with no known risk factors is not covered.

SUBJECT: Food allergy testing and immunization
COVERED: Not covered
EXCEPTIONS: None
REFERRAL: n/a
Co-pay: n/a
CPT CODE: 95075 (Ingestion challenge test)
PROCEDURE:

Food allergy testing and immunization are not considered scientifically proven to be effective and therefore are not covered. This policy also includes testing for systemic Candida infections.

Note: There are several tests for foods included in the standard series of allergy (skin) test performed. These tests will be covered as part of the series but additional testing for food allergies is not covered.

SUBJECT: Bone densitometry (osteoporosis survey)
COVERED: Covered when medically necessary and meets the criteria
                        outlined below.
EXCEPTIONS: Not covered as a general screening exam in the absence
                        of indications listed below.
REFERRAL: Required for HMO; Precertification by Medical
                        Director required
Co-pay: Outpatient services copay; appropriate coinsurance/
                        deductible
CPT CODES: 76075
PROCEDURE:

Osteoporosis is an age-related disorder characterized by decreased bone mass and increased susceptibility to fractures in the absence of other recognizable causes of bone loss. There are two common forms: involutional and secondary. Involutional osteoporosis is the progressive loss of bone mass that occurs naturally with age. Secondary osteoporosis occurs as a complication of a predisposing medical condition (e.g. chronic renal disease, endocrine disorders, malabsorption syndromes, or drug therapy).

Bone densitometry is a covered benefit when the criteria outlined below are met.
CRITERIA:

• In symptomatic (bone pain or suspicious bony abnormality) or known estrogen-deficient female patients for whom the decision to use estrogen replacement therapy depends on information regarding the benefits vs risk of therapy. Post-menopausal status is, in itself, not an indication for this study.

- Monitoring of estrogen therapy patients for baseline studies and follow-up.
- To determine if significant osteoporosis is present when associated with vertebral pain, osteopenia on conventional X-ray, or fracture.
- Evaluation of patients with secondary osteoporosis due to a pre-disposing medical condition such as:
    - chronic renal disease and/or renal dialysis
    - endocrine disorders
    - diabetes mellitus
    - malabsorption syndromes
    - drug therapies (e.g. corticosteroids, anticonvulsants, cancer chemo-therapy, lupron)
- Repeat studies of one site will be covered when used for determining efficacy of therapy. The studies should be performed no more frequently than once yearly.

CONTRAINDICATIONS:

- Bone densitometry is not covered as a routine screening test for osteo-porosis prophylaxis.
- Women who refuse to consider estrogen or other therapy to slow bone loss, or in whom estrogen replacement therapy is contraindicated.
- Members whose work-up treatment will not be altered by bone mass measurements.
- Members already on therapy for whom no additional work-up is con-templated, or in whom no treatment adjustment or substitution of other drugs is possible.
- Members with unequivocal roentgenographic evidence of spinal osteo-porosis or multiple crush fractures, where no therapeutic intervention or change is possible.

Reengineering Sentara

In Chapter 7 reference was made to Sentara Health System's radical reengineering programme aimed at all significant elements of the company.

Sentara's approach went beyond a simple cost-reduction exercise (although cost savings form a major projected benefit – $47.7m by 1997 with annual savings projected of $95m by the year 2000). The current revenue base was about $800 million. Underpinning the restructuring initiative were three key needs:

- to redefine the operating philosophy to maximize the benefits of an integrated system

- to centre the strategic direction on developing the managed care market

- to maintain profitability.

This appendix concentrates on the manner by which Sentara has approached the task of reengineering itself and the implications of such an exercise. In order to set this in context a summary of Sentara's principal operations and the background against which the decision to reengineer was taken are sketched out below. From this it should become apparent that there is a discernible tension between achievement of change as set out above and the maintenance of profits at historical rates of return. Moreover, there may be an underlying strategic crossroads for the company which the reengineering process will make explicit. Specifically, whether Sentara should abandon over time its provider infrastructure and concentrate on the insurance market, and/or assume a for-profit status?

The not-for-profit ethos is considerable within Sentara, particularly as the company has its roots in the local community and charitable care. However, such altruism needs to be financed and the opportunities to generate large operating margins from other payers on a continued basis are open to question. Moreover, the entrepreneurial nature of many of Sentara's executives has already been noted (Chapter 7). This 'spirit' sometimes sits in an uneasy relationship to notions of institutionalized

altruism in a manner not dissimilar to the tensions seen in the NHS since
the arrival of the internal market.

Context

Sentara is an integrated health care company – that is, it contains both
insurance (purchaser) and clinical services (provider) functions. Its range
of functions is not unlike that found within a pre-reorganization health
authority with the important caveat that the managed care component
covers just under 7% of the local population (in 1994 HMO enrolment
was 181 500 out of 1 600 000 insurable lives). Whilst some hospitals'
income is generated from Sentara-insured cases, the majority comes from
patients of other insurers/self pay/government schemes. Profits come from
both sectors but historically by far the greatest component was/is from the
hospitals. In 1994 some 70% of operating revenue came from this sector.
However, the managed care market is growing as can be seen from the fact
that 98.2% of operating revenues came from hospitals in 1982. A fundamental issue resides in the question 'in which sector does the future lie in
terms of maximizing business opportunities/profit'? As in the UK, providers and purchasers perceive themselves as having different interests –
the purchaser (managed care) division wishes to reduce hospital utilization
and costs. Providers wish the opposite. It is not difficult to imagine that
these camps can map out radically different strategic directions for the
company.

In contrast to the NHS, the significant additional dimension in deciding
which course to follow is the profit motive. Whilst the company wishes to
enhance the population's health, improve coverage and lower costs, its
ultimate goal is to generate profits through these actions. This quickly leads
to the question of where most of the profits come from. As previously
noted, the current answer is the hospitals.

US managers and clinicians have been brought up in a culture where the
conventional wisdom is that success is a factor of one's ability in maximizing utilization of the particular service you offer. Company structures
(and Sentara's was no exception) encourage entrepreneurship within this
framework, but are typically highly compartmentalized, both in their
endeavours and their reporting/reward system. In the case of Sentara, its
historical division into de facto separate companies (with their own boards,
targets, accountabilities and bonus schemes) emphasized the competitive
culture but made it difficult to pursue either corporate efficiencies or obtain
the desired leverage associated with an 'integrated health system'.

The company recently replaced the six subsidiary boards with a single consolidated board and has stated that: 'Sentara must shift from being a facility/provider driven organization to a "market driven" organization.' Furthermore, they have agreed 'to focus on managed care while maintaining market leadership in other businesses'.

The willingness and ability to engineer this change, coupled with the wisdom of the strategy itself, will be key in deciding the success of the reengineering programme (against the targets Sentara set itself). The danger is that the exercise may degenerate into a conventional cost-reduction programme as the interests of the hospital sector (and clinicians) reassert themselves – particularly if managed care cannot replicate or enhance absolute and relative profitability. Perhaps the most difficult reengineering task will be to create a system of incentives and rewards that encourage company-wide cooperation without unduly blunting the innovative capacity of executives, in effect creating a win–win situation for both purchaser and provider organizations and the individuals who control them. This is of interest to the NHS where similar tensions reside within the internal market. It should be noted that a win–win situation does not mean a retention of the status quo.

Notwithstanding the internal dynamics of profit maximization, Sentara had to respond to the changing US health care scene. The decision to reengineer both recognizes and is intended to embrace this. Sentara's decision to shift attention from the facilities on which its success has largely been based – its hospitals – is motivated by a knowledge that other companies will increasingly compete for the lucrative Hampton Roads market. These companies may have considerable resources at their disposal. The argument goes that Sentara has shown its competitors the direction that they have to compete – through Sentara's penetration of the managed care market – and it has to continue to lead the change (at the same time anticipating government action) or fall behind. In short, the market is dynamic and requires an appropriate response from Sentara.

This is complicated by the fact that the US health market (and Sentara's geographic centre of operations is no different) has considerable excess capacity. Health care – and the company – has historically bucked the trend of falling prices and reduced profits which would characterize such a 'market'. However, Sentara's stated direction (and the changes indicated at a national level) promote the role of HMOs – for whom the ability to generate profits depends largely on their capacity to minimize utilization of expensive (hospital) services and generally drive costs down. This is further reinforced by Sentara's desire to retain or preferably expand its market share. Given increasing competition, the initial reaction is that this can only be achieved by further squeezes on the hospital sector. Maintaining bottom-line profitability will be a challenge – even with the intended cost-efficiencies – as the typical HMO margins are less than those currently derived from hospitals. Moreover, the more successful the HMO is at recruiting members (through a reputation for low premium/high quality) the fewer other sources hospitals will have to charge differential rates to make up their profit margins. Competition from other HMOs (particularly well resourced ones) can only serve to accentuate that trend.

The difficulties in releasing excess capacity in health care are not dissimilar to the difficulties found in the UK. Closing down hospitals is unpopular with local communities, health professionals and interest groups. Added to this there are the business issues involved in writing off past investments – when you have considerable sums of money invested in fixed assets it may seem that the pain of getting out outweighs the costs of staying in! As in the NHS, there remain formidable barriers to exit. Excess capacity and the impact of fundholders on traditional patterns of funding and service provision are issues for the NHS. Sentara's response, and in particular their reengineering initiative, is pertinent to the way the NHS is tackling (or otherwise) these issues.

The reengineering process

There are features of Sentara's reengineering initiative which are particular to the USA or the company itself and the benefits of describing these are thought too marginal for inclusion, e.g. a review of the cash management policy allowing greater funds to be diverted to the investment portfolio, thus yielding higher rates of return.

The reengineering process was principally driven via four teams with a core membership of around five staff drawn from multidisciplinary backgrounds. Each team had a corporate 'sponsor' (a senior vice-president) whose job was in part to ensure that the process retained senior management commitment and that 'territorial' disputes between reengineering teams and established departments did not occur.

The four teams' remits were broadly as follows:

- customer acquisition (including sales and marketing of all services, the 'products' being offered and how to ensure customer retention)

- care delivery (including hospital, primary, long-term and community care. Particular emphasis on ways of improving patient flow and patient-focused care)

- enablers (including support services: finance, human relations, IT, estate management, supplies)

- 'quick hits' (discrete projects designed to release monies, improve efficiency, e.g. diagnostic services, rationalization).

The latter team had a shorter life-expectancy than the others, and was being utilized for 'value for money' issues aimed at quickly reducing costs/generating revenues.

Reengineering offers an opportunity to start from scratch and redesign work in ways that are more efficient. This means challenging current ways of thinking about how and why things are done. This is the manner in which Sentara has approached reengineering. Contrast this with health authority reorganization where a great opportunity was lost. For example, the All Wales Group looking at IT spent more of its time considering the ownership and transfer of assets than on the use of information systems to streamline work and increase effectiveness. No monies were made available for such initiatives in any case. This reflected a general concern that the principal managerial objective was to manage the transition, not work on ways the new authorities could be more effective.

Reengineering costs money and makes considerable demands on key personnel time and energies. Sentara explicitly took this into account in the following ways:

- the transfer of 28 of some of Sentara's 'best and brightest' staff on a full-time basis to create four reengineering teams. Most of these staff will remain with these teams over a year and certain job guarantees have been given to ensure recruitment and retention of the appropriate staff

- the creation of corporate 'sponsors' for each team and for the overall process amongst the company's vice-presidents and key stakeholders

- capitalization of required changes. Sentara is prepared to invest now for future savings and long-term viability. Its budget for management consultancy alone ran into millions of dollars. In Wales, the Welsh Office position that there be no transitional funding for the creation of the new authorities demonstrated fundamentally poor judgement in this respect

- Sentara is reengineering both as a response to and in an attempt to shape the forces of change within US health care. It wishes to be proactive. This is not without attendant difficulties which, to a degree, would be found in any change process but are accentuated in this most dynamic of industries. The difficulties involved in reengineering include the heavy demands on key staff, and possible failures in communication.

Some Sentara staff regularly work 7.00am to 7.00pm. This was an established part of company culture before reengineering added additional workload and demands for meetings. To an outside observer, current work habits border on the dysfunctional although it would appear that this level of commitment is somewhat the cultural norm for US business. One can, however, question the long-term effects of what may be described as a pressure cooker environment on morale and effectiveness. An important issue is whether Sentara can find a way of 'working smarter' as it has probably reached the point of diminishing returns by the traditional method of working longer hours to achieve objectives. Moreover, it was clear that Sentara management was no more successful in reducing time spent in meetings (many of them standing committees) than the NHS. It found itself locked in the managerial paradox that staff need to create new committees and attend more meetings to decide how ultimately to reduce time spent on meetings!

There is also a constant danger that the left hand (reengineering) will not know what the right hand (operations) is doing and vice versa. An extremely active communications policy is required which has to go beyond newsletters and so on. Sentara has recognized this and has set up a communications group to meet this need. However, it is unlikely that Sentara's world will fit into neat boxes whereby operations make decisions that only impact on the present whilst the reengineering teams retain the strategic overview. This is particularly the case in the information systems arena. Sentara is both an information-dependent and an information-intensive company. Its ability both to utilize and rationalize its information systems is a key issue within the reengineering process. System integration and the development of a company-wide EIS should rank as one of the strategic foundations on which the 'new' company operates. The NHS faces similar challenges and, although Sentara is by no means guaranteed success in this area, it at least demonstrates an appreciation of the gravity of the issue. Those charged with the reorganization of commissioning authorities might wish to reexamine the relative weight being given to these issues as a means of achieving the desired benefits and efficiencies of the 'new' authorities.

Significant change normally requires revision of an organization's culture. This is not achieved overnight. In Sentara's case the traditional mindset was that the hospital business was 'core' and its interests had primacy. As previously outlined, this was being explicitly challenged through the reengineering initiative. Interestingly, although there was a company-wide acceptance of the need to adapt to a changing market, the 'managed care' revolution had not yet materialized. During the six months the author worked with the company, the expectations and language of executives changed subtly. Talk of revolution was replaced by observations that managed care appeared to be evolving gradually, and that maybe it was premature to turn one's back on the more profitable 'indemnity insurance' market. This was articulated by one executive as follows:

> We woke one morning and announced to everybody that henceforward our core business was 'managed care'. The trouble was, you don't change your core business overnight. Our expertise is predominantly the hospital business, our profits are concentrated there – we understand that end of the business. We went off trying to buy ourselves a managed care market and found it wasn't working. We were isolating part of the organisation from economic reality – and it's the worst thing you can do!

A parallel might be drawn with health authorities' proclamations that they are now 'primary-care led' and the balance of attention is with primary not secondary care, preventing illness, not reacting to it, etc.

For Sentara, change was a function of the market – it made changes in anticipation of the market and to try and shape it. If it subsequently had misread the market, then – however painful – it will probably change again. The issue is not whether it is making the right or wrong decisions (which is subject to debate) but that it demonstrates a flexibility which it is difficult to see can be replicated in any system dominated by politics and civil servants.

In conclusion, contrasting Sentara's reengineering initiative with NHS reorganization is instructive. Sentara is attempting to follow the textbook methodology for major change, as prescribed by its management consultants. If they are to be criticized at all it may be for the associated emphasis on following the 'consultancy' line. It is considered likely that as the members of the reengineering teams grow in experience and confidence, they will increasingly seek to cut this expensive umbilical cord. The NHS in contrast seems to be seeking to commit practically every error in the reengineering 'book'. The importance of this observations lies in the fact that both the UK and US health care systems are experiencing rapid change with many similar issues and organizational conflicts. Policy-makers in the UK need to consider what skills and techniques are transferable (in this case with regard to reengineering) and in this context why a business believes that reengineering requires the level of investment described above if it is to prosper, yet the NHS can obtain its objectives with no material investment?

Glossary

Accreditation. Certification by a non-governmental accrediting organization that a given health care provider meets that organization's standards.

Accrual. The amount of money that is set aside to cover expenses. The accrual is the plan's best estimate of what those expenses are, and (for medical expenses) is based on a combination of data from the authorization system, the claims system, the lag studies, and the plan's history.

ACS contract. A contract between an insurance company and a self-funded plan where the insurance company performs administrative services only and does not assume any risk. Services usually include claims-processing, but may include other services such as actuarial analysis, utilization review, etc.

Actuarial. Refers to the statistical calculations used to determine the insured rates and premiums based on projections of utilization and costs for a defined population.

Actuarial assumptions. The assumptions that an actuary uses in calculating the expected costs and revenues of the plan. Examples include utilization rates, age and sex mix of enrollees, cost for medical services, etc.

Acuity level. A means of measuring the level of care required for inpatient and outpatient services.

Administrative services only (ASO). A contractual arrangement to provide administrative services to an employer who sponsors a self-funded health plan. Services may include some combination of claims-processing, actuarial analysis, utilization review and other insurance-related functions. ASOs may be executed by insurance companies or other third party administrators.

Admission certification. A method of assuring that only those patients who need hospital care are admitted. Certification can be granted before admission (preadmission) or shortly after (concurrent).

Adverse selection. The tendency of persons who have poorer than average health expectations to seek or continue comprehensive insurance and participation in managed care programmes to a greater extent than do persons who have average or better health expectations. Increases potential for higher than expected utilization and for costs above budgeted projections.

Any willing provider (AWP). Refers to state laws requiring a managed care organization to accept any physician or non-physician provider who meets the network's usual selection criteria, is willing to be reimbursed at the managed care organization's rates and agrees to the managed care organization's utilization guidelines. HMOs have opposed AWP legislation since they prefer to contract selectively with providers in order to control the quality and efficiency of their network of care.

Balance billing. The practice of charging full fees in excess of the insurer's reimbursable amounts, then billing the patient for that portion of the bill which the insurer does not cover.

Capitation. A method of payment for and charging for health services in which an HMO, medical group, or institution is paid a fixed amount for each person served, usually monthly. The amount of money paid covers services provided regardless of the actual value of those services. Specific service costs are often expressed as dollars per member per month in development of capitation rates and premiums.

Carve-out. Services separately designed and contracted to an exclusive independent provider by a managed care plan. For example, an HMO may 'carve-out' the mental health benefit and select a specialized vendor to provide these services on a stand-alone basis.

Closed panel. A managed care plan that contracts with physicians on an exclusive basis for services, not allowing members to see physicians outside of the limited exclusive panel of providers for routine care. Examples include staff and group model HMOs, but could apply to a large private medical group that contracts with an HMO.

Coinsurance. Form of cost-sharing whereby an insured individual pays a percentage of the cost of covered services.

Community rating. Method of establishing premiums for health insurance. The premium is based on the average cost of actual or anticipated health care used by all enrollees in a geographical area or industry and does not vary for different groups or enrollees or take into account such variables as the group's claims experience, age, sex or health status. Community rating helps spread the cost of illness evenly over all health plan enrollees rather than charging the sick more than the healthy for health insurance.

Community rating by class. A modification of established community rating principles, whereby individual groups can have different rates depending on the composition by age, sex, marital status and industry.

Consultant. Very similar to the position of specialist in the US, consultants have successfully undertaken postgraduate examinations in their chosen specialty. Unlike the USA, hospital consultants are direct employees of trusts and would not normally maintain facilities or practice outside the hospital. They are allowed to supplement their NHS salaries through private practice in their own time. As a result, many have opted for only part-time hospital contracts.

Concurrent review. A form of utilization review in which hospital admissions are reviewed and certified within 24 hours of admission, and are monitored for appropriateness thereafter.

Coordination of benefits (COB). A typical insurance provision whereby responsibility for payment for medical services is allocated between carriers when a person is covered by more than one group health benefit programme. The procedures are also designed to try and ensure that no more than 100% of the costs of care are reimbursed to the patient or paid to the provider(s).

Copayment. Form of cost sharing whereby an insured person pays a specified flat amount per unit of service or unit of time (e.g. $15 per visit, $100 per day) while the insurer pays the remaining costs.

Credentialling. The process whereby a managed care organization obtains and reviews the documentation of individual and/or institutional providers in order to decide whether or not to contract with that provider for the provision of specific health care services to its members. Such documentation includes licensure, certifications, malpractice history, etc. The managed care organization generally reviews the information obtained from the provider and verifies that the information is correct and complete.

Current procedural terminology (CPT) code. Designed by the American Medical Association as a method to communicate, by a five-digit number, specific medical care and services. The numbering system covers the majority of recognized medical services a physician can provide and for which they can be reimbursed. The CPT code is used to report services on the claim form.

Department of Health. A division of the Civil Service headed by the Secretary of State for Health. Responsible for health care in England. In Wales this function falls within the overall responsibility of the Welsh Office. In Scotland it is the Scottish Office, and Northern Ireland has its own Civil Service and ministers (the Northern Ireland Office).

Diagnosis-related group (DRG). A system of classifying patients according to categories of diagnosis which should require very similar programmes of treatment and lengths of hospital stays. DRGs were originally used to determine the amount Medicare reimburses for hospital stays and have subsequently been adopted by many insurers, HMOs and states as a standard contract currency for inpatients. When originally introduced in the 1980s it represented a major shift in reimbursement from payment based on charges for every unit of service provided, to prospective payment for a defined episode of care.

Disease management. A systematic approach to providing care to a population of patients with a given conditon. Stated goals are to improve outcomes and lower costs. Tools include: patient and provider education, guidelines for applying alternative therapies, patient monitoring, outcomes assessment and continuous improvement.

Disease management programme. A radical alternative to the problem of managing drug costs. Some of the larger drug companies are at the forefront of this latest mutation of the 'managed care' concept. At its root is the substitution of the drugs company for the HMO, whereby the company takes a capitated amount per member and it assumes the risk for the cost associated with the clinical management of the patient. The idea has general application but is most often promoted in the management of chronic conditions such as diabetes, asthma and hypertension. At its simplest the idea is that a combination of physician and patient education, high quality primary care and the appropriate use of advanced medications will reduce the need for hospitalization and surgical intervention. The pharmaceutical industry believes it may be better placed to operate managed care programmes than the current protagonists as the current 'system' does not necessarily lend itself to the most effective management of the patient – primarily through ignoring the knock-on effects on other components of the health system of efforts to contain costs in a particular arena, and the accompanying fragmentation of care. It is a fascinating concept and one likely to grow on both sides of the Atlantic, but it is in its infancy at present.

Disenrolment. The process of termination of coverage. Voluntary termination would include a member quitting because he or she simply wants out. Involuntary termination would include leaving the plan because of changing jobs. A rare and serious form of involuntary disenrolment is when the plan terminates a member's coverage against his or her will. This is usually only allowed (under state and federal laws) for gross offences such as fraud, abuse, non-payment of premium or copayments, or a demonstrated inability to comply with recommended treatment plans.

Dual choice. Sometimes referred to as Section 1310 or Mandating. That portion of the federal HMO regulations that require any employer with 25 or more employees residing in the HMO's service area, who pays minimum wage, and who offers health coverage, to offer a federally qualified HMO as well. The HMO must request it.

Experience rating. Method of establishing premiums for health insurance in which a group's premium is based on the demographic characteristics and utilization experience of that particular group.

Explanation of benefits (EOB). A description, sent to patients by the health plan, of benefits received and services for which a health care provider has requested payment.

Family deductible. A deductible which is satisfied by the combined expenses of all covered family members. For example, a programme with a $200 individual deductible may limit a maximum of three deductibles ($600) for the family, regardless of the number of family members.

Family Health Services Authority (FHSA). Until April 1996 the payment and monitoring of 'independent' contractor professions – GPs, dentists, pharmacists and opticians – was undertaken by FHSAs as distinct organizations from health authorities. Therefore, they had the lead role in the development of primary care. From April 1996 the FHSA role is part of the newly created authorities.

Favoured nations discount. A contractual agreement between a provider and a payer stating that the provider will automatically provide the payer with the best discount it provides anyone else. Common between Blue Cross and participating hospitals.

Fundholding. The fundholding scheme was introduced in the 1990 internal market reforms. Its essential characteristic is the devolution of direct purchasing power (and monies) for a range of elective procedures to GPs' practices who satisfy certain requirements (principally a minimum list size). Over time the qualifying criteria have been modified to allow more practices to join (reduced list size criteria, pooling of practices, etc.) and the range of services covered by the scheme gradually extended. As of April1996 there are 32 426 GPs, 16 737 (51.62%) acting as fundholders, responsible for purchasing about 35% of all services (health authorities purchase the rest). In addition to continuing to encourage GPs to become fundholders, the government has introduced a small number of pilot total fundholder initiatives where select practices have been given responsibility for purchasing all services. At present, both partial and total fundholding funding is derived from an analysis of historical activity and is not capitation based.

General practitioner (GP). A doctor (the vast majority of whom now work with other GPs in a practice as partners) responsible for delivering primary care services to a defined population (list). The average list size per GP is around 5400. GPs are independent contractors – that is, they are self-employed, but work for the NHS with payment under terms and conditions defined by a national contract. Three distinctive features of general practice are:

- they have 24 hour, 365 days a year responsibility for the patients on their list and are expected to provide a visit service. Cross cover and locum services are permitted but GPs are responsible for financing such arrangements themselves

- GPs refer patients to secondary services but rarely treat their patients in hospital (except some community hospitals providing rehabilitative, nursing-home-type functions). Hospital care is provided by a consultant and his team

- GPs directly employ/have attached to them a primary care team of workers (see Primary care). There are a number of similarities between GPs and the USA's PCPs.

Health Authority. Prior to 1990 health authorities provided hospital, community and ambulance services for a defined geographical area (typically serving around 250 000 persons) with the FHSA responsible for the independent contractor services – GPs, dentists, pharmacist and opticians. The creation of the internal market left the FHSA role unchanged, but fundamentally changed the role of the health authority. The clinical services contained within each authority were encouraged to apply for self-governing trust status, leaving the authorities with the role as purchasers or 'commissioners' of services on behalf of their populations. They do this principally by placing contracts with trusts for clinical services in a similar manner to the way a managed care organization in the USA ensures services for its members. In April 1996 the Health Authorities Act 1995 will lead to the creation of new authorities through the amalgamation of health authorities and FHSA functions and further consolidation of authorities to create larger commissioning entities (average population size 500 000). This is supposed to be taking place alongside the further development of GP led purchasing through extension of the fundholding scheme.

Health Care Financing Administration (HCFA). The federal agency that oversees all aspects of health financing for Medicare and also oversees the Office of Prepaid Health Care.

Health Maintenance Organization (HMO). An organized system of health care that provides directly or arranges for a comprehensive range of basic and supplemental health care services to a voluntarily enrolled group of persons in a geographic area under a prepayment plan. The term HMO is specifically defined in the Federal HMO Act (P.L.93-222) of 1973 and its amendments.

Health plan employer data and information set (HEDIS). A set of performance measures designed to help employers and other purchasers of health care standardize information and compare health plans. The performance measures cover the areas of quality, access, patient satisfaction, membership, utilization and finance. HEDIS was initially developed in 1991 by the National Committee for Quality Assurance.

Incurred but not reported (IBNR). The amount of money that the plan had better accrue for medical expenses that it knows nothing about yet.

These are medical expenses that the authorization system has not captured and for which claims have not yet been made. Unexpected IBNRs have torpedoed more managed care plans than any other cause.

Indemnity insurance. Typically, this means coverage offered by insurance companies whereby covered persons are reimbursed for specified covered services. Payments may be made to the individual incurring the expense or directly to the providers. The important point is that indemnity relates primarily to payments due to a specific loss (injury, illness) incurred by the insured person.

Independent Practice Association (IPA). An organization that has a contract with a managed care plan to deliver services in return for a single capitation rate. The IPA in turn contracts with individual clinicians to provide the services, either on a capitation basis or on a fee-for-service basis.

Independent Practitioner Organization (IPO). Similar to an IPA, an IPO is an organization of providers, usually physicians, that contracts with a variety of health care plans for a variety of services. Such services may include health care (identical to an IPA), utilization review, etc. The primary differences are that most IPAs contract with one single HMO, where an IPO may contract with multiple types of plans, and IPOs generally do not assume risk.

International Classification of Diseases, 9th Revision, Clinical Modification (ICD-9-CM). The classification of disease by diagnosis, codified into four-digit numbers. Frequently used for billing purposes by hospitals.

Joint Commission on Accreditation of Healthcare Organizations (JCAHO). Private, voluntary accrediting organization for all types of health care organizations. Its focus is the outcome, process and excellence in patient care services.

Lifetime maximum. The maximum dollar amount of health benefits a member can receive while insured or covered under the plan, even if the member's coverage is interrupted or terminated and later reinstated.

Maximum allowable charge (or cost) (MAC). The maximum, though not the minimum, that a vendor may charge for something. This term is often used in pharmacy contracting; a related term, used in conjunction with professional fees is 'fee maximum'.

Mixed model. A managed care plan that mixes two or more types of delivery systems. This has traditionally been used to describe an HMO that has both closed panel and open panel delivery systems.

National Health Service (NHS). The comprehensive provision of health care services, principally funded through general taxation which is available to all UK residents. Services are largely free at the point of use. There are copayment charges for drugs, and dentistry (but 'vulnerable' groups are largely excluded from these). NHS services cover primary, secondary and community care, and ambulance services. As of April 1996 the NHS was organized from 127 health authorities purchasing services from 523 trusts. Annual expenditure stood at £42 billion for financial year 1996/7 (approximately 5.6% of GNP). It should be noted that nursing-home care is means tested and for those covered, purchased through Social Services and therefore falls largely outside the above expenditure.

Oregon Plan. In an effort to control health care costs and provide some medical care for its low income citizens, the State of Oregon initiated the Oregon Medicaid Demonstration Project. After much controversy – among professionals, the public and politicians – the scheme was given approval in March 1993. Under the scheme 688 medical treatments were ranked on the basis of a complex formula that considered efficacy, the seriousness of disease and the prevalence of disease and cost. After the list was developed, Oregon pledged to extend medical care to all of its 360 000 poor citizens, who represent about 12% of the state's population, but treatments below a certain level would not be covered, based on available finances. For example, the initial estimate was that the cut would be made at 568 on the ranking system, making 83% of treatments available. For both its supporters and opponents the Oregon Plan is widely regarded as at the cutting edge of health care rationing due to its comprehensiveness and the process used for determining treatment ranking.

Patient's Charter. An initiative launched in 1992 by the Conservative Prime Minister, John Major, with the stated objective of improving public services. In the case of the Health Service, it consists of a series of guarantees and standards in a number of areas ranging from maximum waiting times for treatment to details on the type of information which should be available to patients and relatives. Since its implementation the Charter has provoked some controversy. Advocates state that it shows a clear commitment of Government to listen to the priorities of the public and provide them with measurable standards on which to judge services. Detractors query the relevance of the targets used, claiming that it diverts resources from more worthwhile areas and leads to raised expectations which cannot in reality be met.

Per diem reimbursement. Reimbursement of an institution, usually a hospital, based on a set rate per day rather than on charges. Per diem reimbursement can be varied by service (e.g. mental health, intensive care unit, etc.) or be uniform regardless of intensity of services.

Per member per month (PMPM). A unit of measure, normally in dollars, computed as dollar amount divided by members (or member months).

Physician–hospital Organization (PHO). Group practice arrangement that occurs when hospitals and physicians organize for purposes of contracting with managed care organizations. These relationships are formally organized, contractual or corporate in character and include physicians outside the boundaries of a hospital's medical staff.

Point of Service Plan. A plan where members do not have to choose how to receive services until they need them. A common example is a simple PPO, where members receive coverage at a greater level if they use preferred providers than if they choose not to do so.

Practice guidelines. Specific, professionally agreed upon recommendations for medical practice used within or among health care organizations in an attempt to standardize practice to achieve consistent quality outcomes. Practice guidelines may be instituted when triggered by specific clinical indicators.

Preadmission review. Review of an elective hospitalization prior to a patient's admission in order to ensure that the services are necessary and that they should be provided in an inpatient hospital setting.

Pre-authorization/precertification. The authorization required by an insurance carrier before the member is eligible to receive maximum benefits for hospitalization and other specific services. With some benefit plans, the member is responsible for obtaining pre-authorization prior to receiving services.

Preexisting condition. A condition that existed, or for which a participant was being treated, before enrolment in a current health plan and for which benefits under the plan are not available or are limited.

Preferred Provider Organization (PPO). A plan that contracts with independent providers at a discount for services. The panel is limited in size and usually has some type of utilization review system associated with it. A PPO may be risk-bearing, like an insurance company, or may be non-risk-bearing, like a physician-sponsored PPO that markets itself to insurance companies or self-insured companies via an access fee.

Premium rate. A monetary amount charged employers or individuals to prepay the cost of health care services. The premium rates may vary by contract type. The premium is a specific contractual amount agreed on by the HMO (or an insurer) and an employer to fix a cost for medical services for employees over an agreed period of time.

Primary care. The delivery of clinical services to people at home, or through a GP's practice – rather than requiring hospitalization. Over time, the role of primary care has extended so that the traditional distinction between primary and secondary (hospital) services has blurred somewhat in certain areas e.g. GPs performing minor surgical or diagnostic procedures in the practice premises. Primary care is generally considered to be well developed in the UK (particularly in comparison to the USA). A GP's practice may be made up as follows: four GP 'partners', one trainee, administrative staff (receptionists, office manager), practice nurse, community nurse, community psychiatric nurse, community midwives and health visitor. Some practices also have physiotherapists, counsellors and social work staff operating from practice premises.

Primary care physician (PCP). An internist, paediatrician, family physician or general practitioner in an HMO who cares for the fundamental health care needs of a patient population. PCPs must coordinate and authorize all medical services, non-emergency hospitalizations, specialty referrals and diagnostic workups for a designated panel of patients in order to maintain appropriate health care utilization and coordination of care. Also referred to informally as a 'gatekeeper'.

Reinsurance. Insurance obtained by an HMO or other carrier from another company to protect itself against part or all the losses incurred in the process of honouring the claims of members or policy-holders. Also referred to as 'stop-loss' insurance. The coverage may apply to an individual claim or to all claims during a specified period for an individual enrollee.

Resource-based relative value scale (RBRVS). A classification system used to reimburse physicians and other providers. The system assigns points to specific services based on required training and skill and expended resources. Fees are calculated according to the points. RBRVS was implemented initially by Medicare to adjust the fees paid to primary care physicians relative to specialists.

Risk. The uncertainty of loss or expense levels due to the inability to project with complete confidence the exact health care needs of the HMO population.

Risk pool. A financial arrangement that spreads the risk of utilization and cost among the participants, generally the insurer, the hospitals and the physicians. The pool may insure against unusually high utilization and costs. The pool also may provide incentives for controlling utilization and costs.

Risk retention. A description of the limitations of financial liability remaining with a major entity to the HMO programme. For example, the HMO may accept all risk to guarantee provision of services to its enrolled population. This risk may be limited by arrangements with reinsurers. Also, the fee-for-service/prepaid medical group may take full risk or limit its risk by contractual arrangements with the HMO corporation.

Second surgical opinions. Utilization control to determine appropriateness of surgery by a second provider source.

Self-funded plan (also called *self-insured plan*). A health plan in which the risk for medical costs is assumed by the employer rather than an insurance company. The employer does not purchase insurance coverage, but may contract with an insurer or third-party administrator to administer the benefits. Under the federal Employee Retirement Income Security Act (ERISA), self-funded plans are exempt from certain state laws and regulations.

Shared risk. In the context of an HMO, an arrangement in which financial liabilities are apportioned between two or more entities. For example, the HMO and the medical group may each agree to share the risk of excessive hospital cost over budgeted amounts on a 50–50 basis.

Specialty risk-pooling. Placing a specialty or group of specialties in their own risk pool. Examples of specialty risk arrangements are capitation, fee-for-service with withhold, discounted charges, a global fee (such as an obstetrical global fee), etc.

Stop-loss. A form of reinsurance that provides protection for medical expenses above a certain limit, generally on a year-by-year basis. This may apply to an entire health plan or to any single component. For example, the health plan may have stop-loss reinsurance for cases that exceed $100 000: after a case hits $100 000, the plan receives 80% of expenses in excess of $100 000 back from the reinsurance company for the rest of the year. Another example would be the plan providing a stop-loss to participating physicians for referral expenses over $2500: when a case exceeds that amount in a single year, the plan no longer deducts those costs from the physician's referral pool for the remainder of the year.

Sutton's law ('Go where the money is!'). The Depression-era bankrobber Willy Sutton, when asked why he robbed banks, is said to have replied: 'That's where the money is'. Sutton apparently denied ever having made that statement. In any event, it represents good advice on determining what needs attention both for a managed care plan and any NHS budget.

Trust. Self-governing NHS trusts were established in the 1990 reforms (which created the internal market). Line accountability to the government is maintained through the chairman and non-executive directors of the board who are approved appointments by the Secretary of State and the chief executives reporting relationship to regional general managers (UK) and directors (Wales, Scotland and Northern Ireland) for the performance of the trust.

Underwriters. Insurance professionals who determine if and on what basis an insurer will accept an application for insurance.

Usual, customary, reasonable (UCR) charges. The maximum amount an insurer will consider eligible for reimbursement under group health insurance plans. Charges are generally based on customary fees paid to providers with similar training and experience in a given geographic area.

Utilization. The extent to which a given group uses specific services in a specific period of time, usually expressed as the number of services used per 1000 members per year. Utilization rates may be expressed in other types of ratios such as per member per month or per member per year.

Utilization review. Evaluation of health care delivery, using objective medical criteria, to ensure that the services are medically necessary, provided in the most appropriate setting and are quality care.

Withhold. An amount owed to a provider but not paid at the time of reimbursement for services. This amount is placed in a risk pool and is divided up at the end of the year if certain utilization goals are obtained. These funds are held over to cover specialists' care, catastrophic situations and cost overruns. The amount of withhold per claim is typically determined as a percentage of the claim payment.

Appendix VIII

Refining current contracts – illustrations

Current contract

Inpatients

Specialty	Emergency			Elective		
	Volume	Tariff	Total £	Volume	Tariff	Total £
General Surgery	1600	1445	2 312 000	800	1340	1 072 000
T&O	1530	1850	2 830 500	610	1080	658 800
ENT	450	1130	508 500	1015	700	710 500

Day cases

Specialty	Emergency			Elective		
	Volume	Tariff	Total £	Volume	Tariff	Total £
General Surgery		–		2000	200	400 000
T&O		–		1625	281	456 625
ENT		–		1550	270	418 500

The future

Inpatients: Contract broken down by DRG with tariffs derived by cost weight. Other case mix measures – chargeable procedures/HRGs could also be used.
General surgery: 1600 emergency and 800 elective cases comprising:

			Emergency	Elective
DRG code	Description	DRG Weight	Volume	Volume
119	Vein and ligation and stripping	0.7767	–	31
158	Anal and stomal procedures w/o cc	0.5935	9	19
162	Inguinal and femoral hernia procedures age >17 w/o cc	0.6691	4	54
167	Apendectomy w/o complicated principal diag. w/o cc	0.8053	75	–
182	Esophagitis, gastroent. and misc. digest. disord. age >17 w cc	0.873	53	5
183	Esophagitis, gastroent. and misc. digest. disord. age >17 w/o c	0.5754	158	16
189	Other digestive system diagnoses age >17 w/o cc	0.6544	22	4
198	Total cholecystectomy w/o cde w/o cc	1.3311	–	14
204	Disorders of pancreas except malignancy	1.0403	36	2
260	Subtotal mastectomy for malignancy w/o cc	0.9415	–	16
262	Breast biopsy and local excision for non-malignancy	0.7095	2	24
336	Transurethral prostatectomy w cc	1.5358	3	14
337	Transurethral prostatectomy w/o cc	0.9272	7	41
Band A		2.0	131	85
Band B		0.7 and 2.0	369	165
Band C		0.7	700	410

Note: In the above example, low volume DRGs are banded together to reduce the administrative load. What is defined in detail against being banded together is ultimately a matter of judgement. Tariff is found by multiplying the DRG weight by cost of DRG = 1.0 cost weight.

Day cases

In this instance the contract is shown broken down by procedure.
General surgery: 2000 cases – total cost £400 000 comprising:

Procedure	Volume	Tariff £	Total £
Endoscopy	180	260	46 800
Sigmoidoscopy	332	240	79 680
Colonoscopy	130	230	29 900
Dilation of anal sphincter	45	220	9900
Haemorrhoidectomy	15	220	3300
Excision/biopsy of breast lesion	210	207	43 470
Repair of inguinal hernia	17	225	3825
Varicose veins stripping/ligation	22	200	4400
Excision/biopsy skin/subcutaneous tissue	190	150	28 500
Lymph node excision biopsy	10	170	1700
Cystoscopy	150	214	32 100
Excision of hydrocele	8	170	1360
Male sterilization	75	120	9000
Circumcision	22	120	2640
Misc. procedures Group A	370	129	47 885
Misc. procedures Group B	139	210	29 190
Misc. procedures Group C	85	310	26 350
Total	2000		400 000

References

1 Secretaries of State for Health (1989) *Working for Patients.* HMSO, London.
2 *The National Health Service and Community Care Act 1990.* HMSO, London.
3 Health Insurance Association of America (1955) *Managed care: a health strategy for today and tomorrow.* HIAA, Washington DC.
4 Stalk J (1990) In: *The New York Times,* 25 November.
5 Macara AW (1995) Whither the NHS? *J Pub Health Med.* 17: 3–5.
6 O'Rourke PJ (1995) *Age and guile beat youth, innocence and a bad haircut.* Atlantic Monthly Press, New York.
7 Clark A (1993) *Diaries.* Weidenfeld and Nicholson, London.
8 Ham C (1994) Where now for the NHS reforms? *BMJ.* 309: 351.
9 *Health Authorities Bill 1996.* HMSO, London.
10 Ham C and Maynard A (1994) Managing the NHS market. *BMJ.* 308: 846.
11 Will AM (1995) Contracting is a recipe for inefficiency. *BMJ.* 310: 60.
12 Ham C and Shapiro J (1995) The future of fundholding. *BMJ.* 310: 1150.
13 Anon (1996) *Fundholding.* 19 June, p. 9.
14 Audit Commission (1996) *What the doctor ordered?* HMSO, London.
15 Shallcross M (1995) Beckett's great balancing act. *Br J Healthcare Management.* 1: 485.
16 Harman H (1996) Labour: substantial work is under way on how to implement the details of our health policy. Letter in *Health Service J.* 106 (5512): 23.
17 Klein R (1996) Labour draft election manifesto. *BMJ.* 313: 68.
18 Deffenbaugh J (1996) Labour saving devices. *Health Service J.* 106 (5512): 27.
19 Warden J (1996) Labour pledges to cut NHS bureaucracy. *BMJ.* 313: 7.
20 Health Management Division, Welsh Office (1996) Letter to Chief Executives (unpublished).
21 Kongstvedt PR (ed) (1995) *The managed care handbook* (3rd edn). Aspen, Maryland.

22 Weiner JP and Ferris DM (1990) *GP budget holding in the UK: lessons from America.* King's Fund Institute, London.

23 Schwartz W and Aaron H (1984) *The painful prescription: rationing hospital care.* The Brookings Institution, Washington DC.

24 Bevan G, Holland W and Mays N (1989) Working for which patients and at what cost? *Lancet.* i: 947–9.

25 Popper C (1995) Do we need an Ofhealth? *BMJ.* **310**: 1618–19.

26 Earl-Slater A, Knight J and Saviour W (1995) Developing a case for OfHealth: a health market's regulator. *Br J Healthcare Management.* **1**: 497–500.

27 Personal correspondence, 1995.

28 Wrightson C and William J (1990) *HMO rate setting and financial strategy.* Health Administration Press Perspectives, Ann Arbor, Michigan.

29 Welsh Office (1996) *A national framework for the provision of secondary care within general practice.* FHSL, Wales.

30 NHS Management Executive (1993) *Costing for contracting, cost allocation, general principles and approach for 1993/94.* HMSO, London.

31 Lutz S (1995) Day of the per diem. *Modern Healthcare: Weekly Business News.* **13 Nov**: 44–8.

32 Welsh Office (1994) *Casemix in contracting, DGM(94)143.* FHSL, Wales.

33 Anon. (1991) *Strategies for casemix management.* Silicon Bridge Associates, Basingstoke.

34 Ham C, Robinson R and Benzeval M (1990) *Health check: health care reform in an international context.* King's Fund Institute, London.

35 Anderson DF and Berlant JL (1995) *Managed mental health and substance abuse services.* In: Kongstvedt PR (ed.) *The managed care handbook* (3rd edn) pp. 150–62. Aspen, Maryland.

36 Anon. (1996) Careless Britain. *The Economist.* **10 August**: 16.

37 Peck E (1995) Mental health and the primary health care team: building bridges. *Primary Care Management.* **5**: 4.

38 Audit Commission (1995) *Finding a place: a review of mental health services for adults.* HMSO, London.

39 Chief Medical Officers of England and Wales (1995) *A policy framework for commissioning cancer services.* HMSO, London.

40 NHS Executive (1996) *Seeing the wood, sparing the trees. Efficiency scrutiny into the burdens of paperwork in NHS Trusts and Health Authorities.* HMSO, London.

41 Little S (1996) Taking the plunge. *Fundholding.* **15 May**: 22.

42 Welsh Office (1995) *GP's out of hours services.* FHSL, Wales.

43 Bogle I and Chisholm J (1996) Primary care: restoring the jewel in the crown. *BMJ.* **312**: 1624–5.

44 Changing Roles Group (1995) *A fresh start*. NHS, Wales.

45 Royce R (1995) Creative tensions. *Health Service J*. **105** (5460): 26.

46 Governance Committee (1995) *To the greater good: recovering the American physician enterprise*. Advisory Board Co, Washington DC.

47 Boland P (1991) *Making managed healthcare work: a practical guide to strategies and solutions*. McGraw Hill, New York.

48 Wolfe S (1992) Quoted in *Medical Economics*. 20 January.

49 Illiych I (1975) *Medical nemesis: the expropriation of health*. Penguin, London.

50 Buck N, Devlin HB and Lunn JN (1988) *The report of a confidential enquiry into perioperative deaths*. Nuffield Provincial Hospitals Trust, King's Fund Institute, London.

51 Anon. (1995) IRC PAS to get fourth new owner in five years. *Health Service J*. **105** (5480): 4.

52 Locke C (1996) What value do computers provide to NHS hospitals? *BMJ*. **312**: 1407–1410.

53 Berliner H (1996) The debate is not academic. *Health Service J*. **106** (5516): 19.

54 Hackler C (1993) Health care reform in the United States. *Health Care Analysis*. **1**: 5.

55 Gregory P (1995) Letter to Chairman and Chief Executives, NHS Wales (unpublished).

56 Powell JE (1976) *Medicine and politics: 1975 and after*. Pitman Medical, Tunbridge Wells.

57 Belasco JA and Stayer RC (1995) *Flight of the buffalo*. Warner Books, USA.

58 Kennedy A (1988) *The rise and fall of the great powers*. Random House, New York.

59 Dix A (1996) Capital gains. *Health Service J*. **106** (5490): 1.

60 Black A (1996) Make PFI a capital idea. *Health Service J*. **106** (5521): 20.

61 Owen JW (1994) Letter to Chairman and Chief Executives (unpublished).

62 Anon. (1995) News section. *Health Service J*. **105** (5482): 4.

63 Griffiths R (1983) *Report of the NHS management enquiry*. DHSS, London.

64 Spiers J (1995) *The invisible hospital and the secret garden: an insider's commentary on the NHS reforms*. Radcliffe Medical Press, Oxford.

65 Saporito W (1992) Why price wars never end. *Fortune*. **25** (6): 68–78.

66 Firshein J (1996) Hospital mergers booming in USA. *Lancet*. **347**: 1688.

67 Cardiology Pre-eminence (1995) *Cardiac capitation: executive briefing.* Advisory Board Co, Washington DC.

68 Weiner JP (1994) Forecasting the effects of health reform on US physician workforce requirements. *JAMA.* **272** (3): 222–30.

69 Yates J (1995) *Private eye, heart and hip.* Churchill Livingstone, Edinburgh.

70 Light D (1996) Betrayal by the surgeons. *Lancet.* **347**: 812–13.

71 McPherson K (1995) How should health policy be modified by the evidence of medical practice variations? In: Marinker M (ed.) *Controversies in health care policies: challenges to practices.* BMJ Publishing, London.

72 Walley T and Barton S (1995) A purchaser perspective of managing new drugs: interferon beta as a case study. *BMJ.* **311**: 796–9.

73 Royce R (1995) The use of outcomes in commissioning: problems and progress. *Br J Healthcare Management.* **1**: 509–12.

74 Orwell G (1950) *Shooting an elephant and other essays.* Harcourt Brace, New York.

75 In: Crichton M (1970) *Five patients.* Arrow Publications, London.

76 Firshein J (1996) 'Do not resuscitate' orders are age limited. *Lancet.* **348**: 353.

77 Royce R (1995) Observations on the internal market: will the dodo get the last laugh? *BMJ.* **311**: 431–4.

78 Klein R (1995) *Priorities and rationing: pragmatism or principles?* *BMJ.* **311**: 761–2.

79 Evans D (1995) Infertility and the NHS. *BMJ.* **311**: 1586–7.

80 Royal College of Physicians (1995) *Setting priorities in the NHS: a framework for decision making.* RCP, London.

81 Oregon Health Services Commission (1993) *Oregon Medicaid Demonstration Project.* OHSC, USA.

Index